Attribution

G. Weary   M.A. Stanley
J.H. Harvey

Attribution

Springer-Verlag
New York Berlin Heidelberg
London Paris Tokyo

Gifford Weary
Department of Psychology
Ohio State University
Columbus, OH 43210, USA

John H. Harvey
Department of Psychology
Spence Laboratories of Psychology
The University of Iowa
Iowa City, IA 52242, USA

Melinda A. Stanley
Department of
Psychiatry and Behavioral Sciences
University of Texas Medical School
at Houston
Houston TX 77030, USA

Library of Congress Cataloging in Publication Data
Weary, Gifford, 1951–
    Attribution.

    1. Attribution (Social psychology)   I. Stanley,
Melinda A. (Melinda Anne)   II. Harvey, John H.,
1943–   .   III. Title.
HM291.W288   1989   302   88-33628
ISBN 0-387-96917-9 (alk. paper)

Printed on acid-free paper

Typeset by Asco Trade Typesetting Limited, Hong Kong.
Printed and bound by R.R. Donnelley & Sons, Harrisonburg, Virginia.
Printed in the United States of America.

9 8 7 6 5 4 3 2 1

ISBN 0-387-96917-9 Springer-Verlag New York Berlin Heidelberg
ISBN 3-540-96917-9 Springer-Verlag Berlin Heidelberg New York

To Grace Heider

Other attribution volumes (e.g., Harvey, Ickes, & Kidd, 1976) have been dedicated to Fritz Heider as the founder of attribution theory. We wish to dedicate the present volume to Fritz Heider's colleague, collaborator, and devoted spouse of over five decades, Grace Heider. We know that Fritz, who died January 2, 1988, would endorse the view that Grace made invaluable contributions to his thinking and writing about attributional processes.

Preface

This book initially was conceived in 1986 by Weary and Harvey as a revision and update of their 1981 *Perspectives on Attributional Processes* (published by Wm. C. Brown, Dubuque, Iowa). However, the extensive nature of recent work on attributional processes and the opportunity to collaborate with Melinda Stanley as a coauthor led to a plan to develop a more comprehensive work than the 1981 book. It definitely is an amalgam of our interests in social and clinical psychology. It represents our commitment to basic theoretical and empirical inquiry blended with the applications of ideas and methods to understanding attribution in more naturalistic settings, and as it unfolds in the lives of different kinds of people coping with diverse problems of living. The book represents a commitment also to the breadth of approach to attribution questions epitomized by Fritz Heider's uniquely creative mind and work in pioneering the area. To us, the attributional approach is not a sacrosanct school of thought on the human condition. It is, rather, a body of ideas and findings that we find to be highly useful in our work as social (JH and GW) and clinical (GW and MS) psychology scholars. It is an inviting approach that, as we shall describe in the book, brings together ideas and work from different fields in psychology—all concerned with the pervasive and inestimable importance of interpretive activity in human experience and behavior.

In this book, our coverage of work on attributional processes has been carefully selected. As in the 1981 book, we have presented in the first two chapters surveys of major foundation work and early qualifications and extensions in the field produced in the 1950s, 1960s, and 1970s. We also have examined more recent critical analyses of these early works. The content of chapter 3 is entirely new to this book. In it we have discussed contemporary theoretical and empirical work on cognitive processes underlying attributional activity. In contrast to the earlier inferential models, the more recent ones rely to a greater degree on an information processing metaphor and, consequently, are concerned with more molecular cognitive processes (e.g., processes of information encoding, representation, memory, causal reasoning). Additionally, in chapter 3 we have examined recent work aimed at elucidating basic perceptual processes underlying attributional activities. Chapter 4 is an update of work (presented by Ben Harris in the 1981 book) on developmental aspects of the causal inference process. In chapters 5–9, we have surveyed applications of attributional analyses. Several of these chapters cover material not found in the earlier book. In particular, we call the reader's attention to chapter 5, which covers attributional processes in close relationships, chapter 6, which examines attribution and health-related functioning, and chapter 9, which surveys the vast literature on attribution and achievement behaviors. We believe that these additions to the book, as well as updated chapters on attributional processes and the development and treatment of maladaptive behavior patterns, represent important complements to the theoretical work covered in the first half of the book.

While the work is indeed the product of a collective effort, Weary is responsible for chapters 1–3, 7, and 8, Stanley for chapters 4, 6, and 9, and Harvey for chapters 5 and 10.

Like its predecessor, this book was written especially for persons who have had some prior interest in the literature on attributional processes and who wish to gain further perspective on this area of work. We have tried to emphasize ideas and approaches that seem to have durability and that will influence in a substantial way the future of attribution theory and research. We have tried to write this book so that it may be used in basic courses and seminars at both undergraduate and graduate levels. Further, we believe that the book may be used as a supplementary source in advanced, and perhaps some introductory, courses in social-personality and clinical psychology that emphasize attribution research.

Finally, we wish to express our thanks to Springer-Verlag for extremely helpful guidance, both in the initiation of the project and along the way as we tried for timeliness but inevitably fell victim to delay created by the demands of our various scholarly loads. Thanks also are due to Faith Gleicher, Bob Jones, Kathy Kost, and Kerry Marsh for their comments on various drafts of chapters. Finally, we express our thanks to Joby Abernathy, Ohio State University, Becky Huber, University of Iowa, and Diana Donnelly, Western Psychiatric Institute and Clinic for help in the typing and production of this work.

June, 1989   Gifford Weary
                                                             Melinda A. Stanley
                                                             John H. Harvey

Contents

Part I Foundations

We interpret other people's actions and we predict what they will do under certain circumstances. Though these ideas are usually not formulated, they often function adequately. They achieve in some measure what a science is supposed to achieve: an adequate description of the subject matter which makes prediction possible (Heider, 1958, p. 5).

Attribution theory in social psychology began with Fritz Heider's (1944, 1958) seminal analyses of how people perceive and explain the actions of others. How one person thinks and feels about another person, how one perceives another, what one expects another to do or think, how one reacts to the actions of another—these were some of the phenomena with which Heider was concerned. It is important to note that his early analyses of social perception and phenomenal causality represent more of a general conceptual framework about commonsense, implicit theories people use in understanding the underlying causes of events they observe in their daily lives, than a set of systematic hypotheses and empirical findings. Perhaps for this reason, the value of Heider's work was not fully appreciated until the mid-1960s, when Edward Jones, Harold Kelley, and their colleagues developed, largely from Heider's ideas, more systematic statements on attributional processes.

During the last three decades, however, theoretical and empirical work on attributional processes has flourished. In fact, between 1970 and 1980, Kelley and Michela (1980) found over 900 published references relevant to attribution. More recently, Harvey and Weary (1984) counted between 400 and 500 relevant papers published between 1978 and 1982. There also has been a string of edited volumes on attribution processes produced during the 1970s and mid-1980s, beginning with the 1972 volume that arose from a 1969 UCLA conference on attribution (*Attribution: Perceiving the Causes of Behavior*, edited by Jones et al.) and including the recent volume by Harvey and Weary (*Attribution: Basic Issues and Applications,* 1985).

Moreover, the reader of this book will observe that attributional analyses have been applied to a number of phenomena. For example, there are attributional analyses of attitude change and persuasion (Wood & Eagly,

1981), helping behavior (Ickes & Kidd, 1976; Meyer & Mulherin, 1980; Weiner, 1980), interpersonal attraction (Hill, Weary, Hildebrand-Saints, & Elbin, 1985; Regan, 1978; Wachtler & Counselman, 1981), equity behavior (Greenberg, 1980), and close relationships (Fincham, 1985b). Attributional analyses also have been applied to coping with diverse physical illnesses (Kiecolt-Glaser & Williams, 1987) and to the development and maintenance of various emotional or psychological problems such as helplessness and depression (Abramson, Seligman, & Teasdale, 1978), loneliness, and shyness (Anderson & Arnoult, 1985). These applications illustrate the potential breadth of theorizing about people's making causal inferences and forming impressions of others across a variety of social settings.

The volume of production in this area and its solid intellectual basis indicate the central importance of attribution work to contemporary psychology. More importantly, at least for the purposes of this book, it indicates that the attribution area is a dynamic and rapidly changing one. In the first part of the book we will attempt to chart the early theoretical foundations, as well as later theoretical qualifications and extensions. We also will examine recent theoretical advances concerned with basic perceptual and cognitive processes involved in attribution. While these discussions will focus on the causal inference processes of adults, the last chapter in this part will examine evidence relevant to the attributional activity of young children and to the specification of developmental patterns in the process of attributing causality, responsibility, and blame.

1
Introduction to Basic Attribution Theories

While this book is about perspectives on attribtion theory and research and while we at times will refer to "attribution theory," we would like to point out that there is no monolithic theory in this domain of work. As soon will become evident to the reader, there are no well-accepted, singular sets of assumptions or hypotheses, nor are there general conclusions concerning attribution processes that are tied together in a coherent logical network. Rather, there are several theoretical approaches to causal attribution processes, each of which has some similarities to and differences from the others. In addition to these attribution conceptions which are concerned primarily with the process of making an attribution, there are a number of analyses that are concerned primarily with the consequences of arriving at a given attribution. Kelley (1978) has termed these latter analyses attributional theories and has commented, "That's what most of the research is about—attribution-based theories of emotion, achievement, motivation, affiliation, helping, revenge, equity" (p. 375). Indeed, we have already noted the diverse and extensive phenomena to which attribution conceptions have been applied. In the first section of this book we will examine attribution theories, and in the next section we will focus on attributional theories; however, the reader should not be misled into believing that there is more theoretical coherence in this area than there really is.

In the section below, we will inquire further about the definition of attribution and about why attributions are made. Next, we will review early basic attribution analyses provided by Heider (1958), Jones and Davis (1965), and Kelley (1967). Other important work on basic attribution processes has been done by Bem (1967a, 1967b, 1972) and also will be reviewed.

Definition and Central Features

What is a causal attribution? An attribution is an inference about why an event occurred or about a person's dispositions or other psychological states. As we shall discuss later in this chapter, we may make attributions about our own dispositions and experiences just as we make attributions about others. Hence, attributions may be perceptions and inferences about others or about self.

As a way of illustrating the meaning of this concept, consider a situation in which two people have just met at a party and are subtly probing whether or not they want to get to know one another further. The male says that he has just broken off a 2-year relationship with a female. He says that he terminated the relationship because (a) she was too dependent on him, (b) he could not take his eyes off other females, (c) they had very different hygienic habits, and (d) he did not get along with her parents. The male's stated reasons for breaking off the relationship are all attributions. They are *perceived causes of behavior*. But it is interesting to note that the female listening to the male probably is forming attributions about the male's conduct—"Did he really do it for that reason? I think that she broke it off and that he was more involved with her than he admits"—and about the other female—"What were her reasons for leaving him? Perhaps she found him to be too selfish, too emotionally distant?"

What do we mean when we say that something is the *cause* of an event? Throughout this book, we will define the cause of an event as that antecedent, or set of antecedents, that is sufficient for the occurrence of the effect. Since we are concerned here with interpersonal events, the cause generally will involve human agency, or the idea that the effect was produced by volitional human actions (Shaver, 1985). Further, we are concerned mostly with perceived causes of such events. The real causes of interpersonal events may be numerous and only partially understood. In our example, then, the cause of the relationship breakup, at least from the perspective of the male, was the set of antecedent conditions identified by him. The effect, of course, was the breakup, an effect over which he had some control.

In addition to forming causal attributions, both persons in our example are forming impressions of one another. This process of impression formation represents an integral part of attributional phenomena, namely, making *dispositional attributions*. These are inferences about what a person is like. Undoubtedly, the female has formed certain impressions of the male's personality based upon his description of his ill-fated romance. But suppose that in the course of the discussion, our female says that she likes to parachute out of airplanes, practice karate, and do pistol target-shooting. It is likely that her comments about her preferred activities also will tell the male a lot about her dispositions or personality characteristics.

When and why do people make attributions? We know that people do make attributions in various situations. When a perceiver sees a stimulus person take an action, the perceiver may well be concerned with more than simply registering observable events. In our example of the two people who have just met at a party, the female may not be content simply to register the male's stated reasons for the breakup of his relationship.

Rather, she may want to know whether he still cares for the other female why he might have mentioned the ill-fated relationship, whether he has difficulty relating to all females, and whether he would have difficulty relating to her. That is, our female may be motivated to understand, or make dispositional inferences about, the underlying nature of the male with whom she is interacting. This need to understand, organize, and form meaningful perspectives about the myriad events people observe every day is considered to be a major goal of attributional processes (Kelley, 1967, 1972b). Without such an understanding of our social world, events would be unpredictable and uncontrollable.

The notion that control motivation is an important instigator of attributional activity recently has achieved indirect and direct empirical support. It has been shown, for example, that aspects of the stimulus information that would be expected to arouse control motivation, such as unexpected information (Clary & Tesser, 1983; Hastie, 1984; Pyszczynski & Greenberg, 1981; Wong & Weiner, 1981) and negative outcomes (Harvey, Yarkin, Lightner, & Town, 1980; Wong & Weiner, 1981), stimulate attributional analyses. Similarly, if the perceiver's involvement (e.g., anticipated future interaction) with or outcome dependency upon a target is great, then it is more important for the perceiver to understand the target person's behavior and hence more important for the perceiver to engage in causal analyses (Berscheid, Graziano, Monson, & Dermer, 1976).

In a direct test of the control motivation hypothesis, Pittman and Pittman (1980) found evidence that attributional activity increases following an experience with lack of control. In their procedure, subjects received one of three levels of helplessness training (none, low, or high) and then read an essay under three sets of attribution instructions (the writer prepared it for pay, the writer did not prepare it for pay, no information given about why the writer had written the essay). The authors found that the attribution variation had greater impact on subjects' judgments about the causal influences on the writer when they had experienced low or high control deprivation; subjects who had had no experience with helplessness did not show judgment differences as a function of the attribution manipulation.

How do people make attributions that render their experiences understandable, controllable, and predictable? Do they rationally process information and then report reasonable, objective inferences? Do they try to explain events in a light that is more flattering to themselves than would be warranted if a more objective account were rendered? Evidence suggests that each of these processes represents a viable base for attributions. But when one process will be operative and the other relatively inoperative is far from clear. Furthermore, there are no doubt mechanisms that govern attributional activity that have not been specified in previous work. Finally, we simply do not know enough about the situations in which people actually engage in attributional activity versus those in which they do not, nor do we know much about different types of attributions (e.g., causal, disposi-tional, responsibility) for different situations. Therefore, let the reader be-ware: The topic of attribution is popular and has been well-researched, but there are many significant questions that remain to be answered in the future.

In the remainder of this chapter we will discuss early theoretical works that have formed the foundation for the development of attribution theory and research.

Attributional Aspects of Heider's Commonsense Psychology

Heider's (1944, 1958) theoretical statements provided the seed for the de-velopment of the attribution area in social psychology. Before the publica-tion of Heider's 1958 book *The Psychology of Interpersonal Relations*, there had been few attempts to conceptualize systematically how people perceive and interpret the actions of others. Heider analyzed in detail how people go about answering questions such as: "Did she intend to hurt him by that action?" "What is he really like when you get to know him?" Heid-er referred to his analysis as "common-sense psychology" or the "naive analysis of action" because he was concerned with the events that occur in everyday life for most people and the manner in which people understand these events and explain them in "commonsense" terms. He described his approach in this way: "Our concern will be with 'surface' matters, the events that occur in everyday life on a conscious level, rather than with the unconscious processes studied by psychoanalysis in 'depth' psychology. These intuitively understood and 'obvious' human relations can, as we shall see, be just as challenging and psychologically significant as the deep-er and stronger phenomena" (1958, p. 1). We should emphasize, however, that in no sense did Heider's analysis represent a naïve conception. Rather, it is an extremely provocative and perceptive theoretical analysis of human social behavior. Researchers have yet to probe adequately many of the eminently researchable ideas contained in Heider's 1958 book.

Heider's Causal Analysis of Perception

At the very heart of Heider's analysis is the view that many principles that underlie person perception have parallels in the field of nonsocial, or object, perception. In *The Psychology of Interpersonal Relations* (1958), Heider presents a comprehensive formulation of the naive, implicit princi-ples that underlie the perception of social objects, "Principles that connect the stimulus configurations presented to a person with his apprehension of them" (p. 21). In other words, his causal description of perception regards the phenomenally given, immediate presence of the objects of perception as the end product of a process. This process may be causally structured into steps.

The initial step in the perception of social objects involves the person toward whom the perceiver's attention is directed. This other person, with his/her psychological processes such as intentions, dispositions, and emotions, is referred to as a *distal stimulus*. Because the distal stimulus is external to and does not directly impact upon the perceiver, information about the distal object (i.e., the person as the object of perception) must be obtained through some form of mediation involving physical stimuli (e.g., light and sound waves). In the case of person perception, the mediation conveys information about the personality of the other as revealed by his/her behavior or from verbal descriptions of the stimulus person's actions made by a third party. The resulting stimulus pattern, or "raw material," with which the perceiver comes into direct contact has been termed the *proximal stimulus*. It is through the mediation that the perceiver and the objects of perception may be said to be causally connected.

The final step in the causal analysis of perception comprises the constructive process within the perceiver that results in the phenomenal percept of the person as experienced by the perceiving organism. In this constructive part of the process, the proximal stimulus may be actively interpreted against a background of subjective forces such as past experiences, wishes, needs, and future expectancies. Percepts will arise that best fit the stimulus conditions and internal systems of evaluations or meanings.

This constructive phase of the perceptual process suggests a hierarchical process ". . . in wich the proximal stimulus gives rise to more peripheral meanings, which in turn play the role of data for the higher levels of construction" (Heider, 1958, p. 44). Heider does not, however, argue that this process proceeds in a one-way fashion from proximal stimulus to more central processes (e.g., logical analysis of information, memory processes, belief systems) in the brain. Rather, he suggests that there is an interaction between the central processes and that the former determines, in some instances more and in some instances less, how the proximal stimulus is organized and, consequently, how the final percept is phenomenally experienced. That is, in some cases causal information may be inherent in the perceptual organization of information as determined by the properties of the perceptual apparatus (Heider, 1959). In other cases, however, causal information may arise from more deliberative, inferential processes within the perceiver.

According to Heider's analysis of social perception and phenomenal causality, then, attribution processes are inextricably intertwined with perceptual processes and are oriented toward the search for structure or dispositional properties. In this analysis, people are seen as trying to develop organized, meaningful perspectives about the numerous events that they observe every day, for it is only ". . . by referring transient and variable behavior and events to relatively unchanging underlying conditions" (Heider, 1958, p. 79) that individuals can predict and control their environments.

While Heider draws many parallels between the principles underlying social and nonsocial perception, he also admits that there are some differences. He believes, for example, that constancy and invariance (always seeing the person as displaying the same traits) in social perception is not as perfect as it is in nonsocial perception. As an illustration, there is some evidence that a perceiver may tend consistently to attribute a stimulus person's behavior to the person (i.e., to stable personality features of the person) regardless of the situation in which the behavior occurs (see the discussion of actor–observer differences, chap. 2). But Heider's analysis would allow for the possibility that a perceiver *may learn* to view others as responding in differentiated ways in different situations. Thus, a mother may learn to view her son as quiet and obedient at home but difficult to manage at school.

Internal Versus External Causal Attribution

Heider (1958) suggests that people search for the causal structure of events via reliance upon attributions to the environment (*external attribution*) or to something in the person involved in the event (*internal attribution*). Types of external attributions include those made to the physical and social circumstances surrounding the action, while types of internal attributions include those to the actor's ability, motivation, attitude, or emotional state. For example, a teacher may conclude that a student's academic problems in school can be traced to the student's difficult family situation. This conclusion represents an external attribution. On the other hand, an internal attribution would be represented by the teacher's inference that the student's problems could be traced to the student's lack of motivation in studying and working hard to comprehend the subject matter. Of course, the teacher may arrive at the conclusion that some mix of these internal and external factors caused the student's problems.

Conditions of Action

Heider (1958) proposed that an action outcome depends upon a combination of environmental force and personal force. *Environmental force* was conceived to refer to important external factors such as the difficulty of a task. *Personal force* was conceived to involve ability, motivation, and intention. Heider suggests that the two necessary and sufficient conditions for the production of an outcome are "can" and "trying." He theorized that the specific components of "can" are, on the one hand, ability and power and, on the other hand, environmental factors. If a person's ability exceeds the difficulty of the task, then we say that he or she "can" produce an effect. Whether or not the effect will be produced then depends on the "trying" component of personal force. "Trying," according to Heider, has both a directional component (what a person intends to do) and a quantitative component (how hard the person is trying to do something). Heider argued that intention is often taken as the equivalent of wishing, or wanting. If, for example, we know that a person is trying to write a book, we usually assume that he or she wants to do it.

In his naive analysis of action, Heider (1958) posited that exertion varies directly with the difficulty of the task and inversely with the power or ability of the person. An implication of this point is that the less power or ability individuals have, the more they will have to exert themselves to succeed; also, the greatest exertion will be needed when individuals have little power or ability and the task is difficult. This analysis also has implications for the extent to which power or ability will be attributed to a person. For example, great power or ability will be attributed to people if they are able to solve difficult tasks with little exertion. As we can see from this discussion of Heider's naive analysis of action, then, our perception of whether individuals have a particular ability or display motivation in certain situations is important. It may affect our understanding of their actions, our predictions regarding their future behaviors, and our attitudes toward them.

Sometimes it is very clear in the absence or failure of action whether it is the "can" or the "try" that is the missing condition. However, in some circumstances the data are sufficiently ambiguous so that the person's own needs or wishes determine the attribution. As an example of such self-serving attributions, Heider (1958) cites the case of the thief who, having no opportunity to steal, considers himself an honest man. In reality, the thief does not steal because the "can" is lacking; he has had no intention to steal and thus is able to claim credit for being law-abiding. Heider also contends that the actions of others provide a fertile field for the influence of the perceiver's needs and wishes on attributions. For example, we may think erroneously that another person is able and intends to do something just because we wish it to happen. In general, Heider contends that erroneous judgments are made when the conditions of action are only partially given or when motivational influences distort the causal inference process. The topic of motivational aspects of attributional activities constitutes a major strand of research in contemporary attribution work; and we will devote considerable attention to it in subsequent chapters of this book.

Causal Versus Responsibility Attributions

"Why did this event happen?" "How much was a specific person responsible for its occurrence?" While questions of causation and responsibility surely are related, they also are conceptually distinct. An individual may be judged as responsible and, hence, as answerable for an event even though he or she did not directly produce it. To take a prototypical example, President Reagan may be held responsible for the Iran-Contra affair even though he apparently had no knowledge of the actions taken by his subordinates.

As we have seen, Heider's (1958) naive analysis of action specified two antecedent forces that jointly cause action outcomes: personal and environmental force. Personal force involves "can" and "trying," while environmental force involves features of the environment such as task difficulty or luck. In Heider's analysis, "can" and "trying" are viewed as the two necessary and sufficient conditions of purposive action.

In contrast to inferences about causality, judgments of responsibility require the consideration of a number of different dimensions. Causality is only one of these dimensions. In general, attributed responsibility to a person will increase with increases in the person's (a) observed or apparent causal contribution to the outcome, (b) knowledge of the consequences of the action taken, (c) intention to produce the outcome, (d) degree of volition versus coercion, and (e) appreciation of the moral wrongfulness of the action (Shaver, 1985). While much of our discussion in this book will focus on questions of causality, a substantial body of literature has been devoted to responsibility attributions. We will review some of this work in chapter 4.

Concluding Points

Heider's main contribution to attribution theory is his conception of the processes and variables involved in a person's attribution of causality. Heider suggests that people operate very much like quasi scientists in their attributional activities. They observe an event and then, often in a logical, analytical way, attempt to discover the connections between the various effects and possible causes. Heider does not argue that people are always objective and rational in their behavior. He points out that sometimes people make attributions that are not based on enough information, that are not based on an adequate analysis of information, or that are distorted by psychological needs and motivations.

This review of Heider's analyses of social perception and the causal inference process has revealed only a small part of Heider's contribution to contemporary attribution work. His work has been and continues to be a profound stimulus for ideas about attributional behavior (see *Fritz Heider: The Notebooks*, edited by Benesch-Weiner, 1988).

Jones and Davis's and Jones and McGillis's Theory of Correspondent Inferences

Jones and Davis's (1965) theory of *correspondent inferences* was the first explicit hypothesis-testing formulation in the area of attribution. This theory set the stage for an upsurge in the amount of research investigating attributional problems. The theory of correspondent inferences basically is concerned with factors that influence an observer's attribution of intent and disposition to another person. It does not explicitly address the question of how individuals understand their own intentions and dispositions.

To analyze the process of making correspondent inferences about others, Jones and Davis employ attributional principles adopted from Heider. In this formulation, a correspondent inference is an inference about individuals' intentions and dispositions that follows directly from or corresponds to their behaviors. If, for example, Jim makes a sarcastic remark to his wife Sally, leading to much emotional distress on the part of Sally, we may infer that Jim is hostile toward Sally and intends to abuse her verbally (our attribution of Jim's intent follows directly from his behavior). We may also make the dispositional inference that Jim's sarcastic remark was not intentional and that he means Sally no ill will; to infer malicious intention here would not be a correspondent inference. But how do we decide whether Jim intended to harm Sally and indeed is a rather malicious person? After all, the couple may have had a long history of marital conflict, and the remark may be interpreted mainly in the context of that history of conflict. Jones and Davis have analyzed a number of factors that might help us make this decision.

Desirability of Outcome and Correspondent Inferences

Jones and Davis (1965) view the cultural desirability of behavior as an important determinant of the attribution of intent and disposition. According to these theorists, behavior that is unexpected, or low in desirability, will be more informative to the perceiver and more conducive to a correspondent inference than will behavior that is expected, or high in desirability. "Correspondence" in attribution often is operationally defined in terms of how confident the attributor can be in making an inference. In our example of Jim and Sally, we may feel very confident in inferring that Jim is generally rather malicious if his remark was not appropriate for the situation in which it was made. That is, if Jim had made his sarcastic remark to his wife at a cocktail party in front of several of his wife's friends, we likely would feel more confident in our attribution of malicious intention than if he had been sarcastic during a heated argument that had occurred in his office. In the former situation, Jim's sarcastic behavior toward his wife would be seen as unexpected and socially undesirable and hence would tell us something about Jim's true nature.

A classic study by Jones, Davis, and Gergen (1961) provides evidence about the prediction that behavior that is low in social desirability for a particular role (out-of-role behavior) will be more informative to a perceiver than will behavior that is high in social desirability (in-role behavior). In this experiment, subjects heard tape recordings of a person presumably interviewing for a job as a submariner or of a person interviewing for a job as an astronaut. Prior to listening to the taped interview, subjects were given descriptions of the ideal characteristics of candidates for the job. For example, subjects expecting to listen to an interview for the astronaut's job were told that the ideal astronaut is a person who is essentially inner-directed (a person who is autonomous and who can get along well without interaction with others); subjects expecting to listen to an interview for the submariners's job were told that the ideal submariner is a person who is essentially other-directed (a person who is gregarious and who likes frequent contact with others). In the actual interview, the job candidate, who was thought to understand the requirements for the job, either acted out of line with the requirements for the job (e.g., acted gregarious and other-directed in the case of the astronaut's position) or acted in line with these requirements. Subjects then were asked to give their impressions of the person with reference to several traits and were asked how confident they were in their impressions.

Jones et al. found that subjects made more extreme judgments and were more confident about them in the out-of-role condition (where the behavior was unlikely to have been caused by the interview situation) than in the in-role condition (where the behavior could plausibly have been caused by the interview situation). For example, subjects reported that they felt strongly and confidently that the astronaut interviewee was an affiliative, nonindependent type of person when he acted in that manner despite the nonaffiliative, independent nature of the job (in a sense, the out-of-role person was seen as breaking out of the constraints of the situation to show his true self).

Noncommon Effects and Correspondent Inferences

A second important determinant of correspondent inferences is the non-common effects associated with an action. Noncommon effects represent distinctive outcomes that follow from an act. Only a few studies have been done to investigate this variable (e.g., Ajzen & Holmes, 1976; Newtson, 1974; Wells & Ronis, 1982). How the variable works in the attribution process may be shown by an example concerning a person who has chosen an alternative from a set of alternatives.

Let us suppose that we are interested in why Jennifer decided to go to college at the University of Kansas rather than Ohio State University. We may analyze the decisional situation and determine that there are a number of common effects associated with Jennifer's choice. For example, both schools are in the Midwest. Both are state schools. Educational opportunities are about the same at both schools. Both schools are coeducational. Tuition at the two universities is about the same. What about noncommon effects? A major one that may tell us something about Jennifer is that Ohio State University has more than twice the number of students than the University of Kansas has. This one noncommon effect may be very informative in helping us understand Jennifer's choice; in a more confident fashion, we may make an inference about Jennifer's dispositions. We may infer confidently that she is not overly assertive and that she fears large classes where it may be difficult for her to interact with her professors. As this example shows, the fewer the noncommon effects associated with an act, the more likely a correspondent inference will be made. If the choice alternatives differ in countless ways, it will be difficult for the perceiver to infer much about the stimulus person based on the decision made.

Personalism, Hedonic Relevance, and Correspondent Inferences

Correspondence of inferences may also be affected by the perceiver's motivational concerns. The effects of an action are said to have *hedonic relevance* for the perceiver if the perceiver is benefitted or harmed by the observed action. An act may be hedonically relevant for the perceiver and yet the perceiver may conclude that the consequences of the action were unintended. Alternatively, if the perceiver concludes that the observed action was uniquely conditioned by his or her presence (i.e., that the positive or negative consequences of the action were intended), inferences may be influenced by the variable of personalism. According to Jones and Davis (1965), the more hedonically relevant and/or personalistic an act is for the perceiver, the more likely the perceiver will be to infer that the act reflects a particular intent or disposition. For example, a negative act intentionally directed toward a particular perceiver is more likely to elicit an inference of malevolent intent than is the same act directed toward another person. (See Enzle, Harvey, & Wright, 1980, for a test of this notion.)

Despite the potential importance of hedonic relevance and personalism in attributional activities, Jones and Davis paid relatively little attention to the role of motivation in their theory of correspondent inferences. Instead, these theorists focused mainly on the more "rational" aspects of the causal inference process. In the next section, we will review briefly a recent reformulation of Jones and Davis's conception.

Jones and McGillis's Analysis

Jones and McGillis (1976) extended and refined major aspects of Jones and Davis's (1965) formulation. As noted above, Jones and Davis originally proposed that an important determinant of the correspondence of inferences is the extent to which behavioral effects fit the perceiver's prior expectation about what most people desire (i.e., the social desirability of behavioral outcomes). In their analysis, Jones and McGillis suggested that this determinant be refined in such a way that effects are assumed to have valences ranging from -1 to $+1$. A maximally desirable effect would have a valence of $+1$, indicating the highest probability that an individual (and most individuals) would want to obtain that effect. Conversely, a maximally undesirable effect would have a valence of -1, indicating the highest probability that an individual (and most individuals) would desire to avoid that effect. According to Jones and McGillis, and consistent with Jones and Davis's (1965) earlier formulation of correspondent inference theory, if a particular person pursues an act having a low valence outcome, we should learn more about that person (with a maximum information gain for a -1 outcome) than if the person pursues an act having a high valence. In other words, the more unexpected a given act, the more informative the action is concerning the underlying dispositions of the person.

Jones and McGillis also suggested that the concept of expected valence applies to a second type of expectancy: the perceiver's prior expectations concerning what effect a *particular* actor desires. This latter type of expectancy might be based upon prior knowledge about the actor. A correspondent inference (or information gain) would then constitute a shift in expected valences so that the target person is seen as desiring certain consequences more or less than before the behavioral observation. For example, suppose we observe someone make a series of speeches favoring personal freedom and autonomy, and subsequently observe the same individual make a speech calling for legal prohibitions against the sale and/or use of marijuana. This later speech would disconfirm our prior expectations about this particular actor and would result in more correspondent inferences regarding this actor's beliefs about the deleterious effects of marijuana than if the later speech had merely confirmed the actor's already demonstrated proautonomy beliefs.

It is important to note that when the expected valence notion is extended to include expectations based upon an individual's prior behaviors, then correspondent inference theory permits analysis of a perceiver's observation over a period of time. This revision of correspondent inference theory by Jones and McGillis (1976) is important because Jones and Davis's (1965) original formulation was concerned only with a single behavioral episode; there was no provision for inferences following more extended experience with a given person. Indeed, Jones and McGillis note that Jones and Davis's ". . . paper might better have been subtitled 'From Acts to Intentions' than 'From Acts to Dispositions'. A disposition is inferred when an intention or related intentions persist or keep reappearing in different contexts" (1976, p. 393). Consequently, the shift from assumed social desirability to assumed valence makes it possible to treat correspodence of inference at any stage in a behavioral sequence.

Another theoretical refinement introduced by Jones and McGillis is the notion of skepticism. As the discrepancy between what the perceiver expects to occur and what actually occurs increases, the perceiver is likely to become skeptical regarding the knowledge gained. For example, Jones, Worchel, Goethals, and Grumet (1971) found that perceivers tended to make rather neutral (i.e., noncorrespondent) attributions regarding a black person's attitude when the person did not vote for a candidate favoring affirmative action. In this study, perceivers presumably found the black person's voting record discrepant from what they expected and, consequently, viewed with skepticism the information gained about the person's attitude.

A review by Deaux (1976) of the literature concerned with attributions for male and female success and failure demonstrates further how expectations can influence the correspondence of dispositional inferences. Deaux concluded from her review of the evidence that for a wide range of tasks, the success of men and the failure of women are more expected and tend to be attributed to ability. However, the unexpected failure of men and the unexpected success of women tend to be attributed to situational factors. Zuckerman (1979) arrived at the same general conclusion as Deaux in his review of the evidence relevant to attributions for unexpected task performance: unexpected outcomes are attributed less to ability and more to situational factors such as luck.

Concluding Points

Jones and McGillis, (1976) introduce other new concepts; these concepts relate especially to how perceivers use their unique experiences with particular individuals and their general experiences with categories of persons to infer the attitudes of stimulus persons. But, in general, Jones and Davis's (1965) and Jones and McGillis's (1976) correspondent inference theory represents a rational baseline model of the causal inference process; Jones and colleagues present a conception of the perceiver as a rational person who evaluates information and makes logical inferences about others. Jones et al. have focused less on the question of how a perceiver's needs, wishes, and motives influence attributions. However, they have suggested that their theory may serve as a model or norm to identify and study attributional biases. As noted in our discussion of Heider, ego-defensive processes no doubt are at work in attributional phenomena, and increasingly they have become a topic for active research and theoretical analyses. Finally, in these theoretical statements, Jones and colleagues have focused mainly on person perception (or attribution to others) as opposed to self-perception. As we will see below, Kelley, and particularly Bem, have made contributions to understanding self-perception and attribution. Nonetheless, to date, the work by Jones and colleagues represents the most systematic, productive, and long-term program of work on processes involved in attribution to others.

Kelley's Contributions to Attribution Theory

Kelley's (1967) review and analysis gave attribution theory and research much stimulation and an integrative approach to understanding both attribution to others and to self. Unlike Jones and colleagues, Kelley assumes that his concepts apply equally as well to self-perception as they do to person perception.

Analysis of Variance (ANOVA) Model of Attribution

Kelley (1967) theorized that people often make causal attributions as though they were analyzing data patterns by means of an analysis of variance (ANOVA), a statistical technique used to determine whether variance on a dependent variable of interest (i.e., the extent to which subjects' scores on a dependent variable differ by condition) exceeds what would be expected by chance. This technique indicates whether an independent variable, such as the home background of a student, had a significant effect on a dependent variable, such as performance in the classroom. In terms of attribution processes, the attributor is assumed to attribute effects to those causal factors (the independent variables in this ANOVA analogy) with which they *covary*, or with which they are correlated, rather than to those from which they are relatively independent. For example, we might want to know if a student's classroom performance uniquely covaried with home and background factors (and, hence, is attributable to these factors), or if it covaried just as much with other factors such as the learning ability of classmates. The principle of covariation between possible causes and effects is the fundamental notion in Kelley's (1967) attributional approach. In Kelley's formulation, the important classes of possible causes are persons, entities (things or environmental stimuli), and times (occasions or situations).

How can attributors know that attribution of a particular effect to a particular cause is valid? According to Kelley, attributors use three types of information to verify whether they have correctly linked causes and effects. These types of information are the distinctiveness, consistency, and consensus associated with the possible causes. To illustrate the meaning of these types of information, consider an attributor's problem in evaluating why a particular employee in a business frequently was involved in dissension and quarreling with other employees. Kelley's (1967) analysis suggests that the attributor may assess how distinctive the employee's behavior is by asking the question, "Does the employee quarrel with other people in other situations (e.g., at home or in relating to neighbors)?" If so, the behavior is not distinctive and the attribution of causality for the conflict most likely would be directed toward the employee (e.g., his/her unfriendly disposition) as opposed to other people or aspects of the work situation.

How does the attributor use consistency information? If the employee argued and was at odds with others consistently over a period of time and with reference to different issues, then the behavior would be consistent over time and modality, and, again, an attribution to the employee's disposition probably would be made. Consensus information would be used to determine whether others also engaged in considerable quarreling at the employee's place of business. If arguing and bickering were commonplace, the attributor might be less likely to attribute the employee's behavior to some personal characteristic. The attributor might guess that conditions at the business were generally unsatisfactory to the employees. On the other hand, if others did not quarrel often, a dispositional attribution would be warranted. In sum, Kelley's (1967) analysis would predict that an attribution to the employee's personal dispositions would be made if the behavior in question was low in distinctiveness, high in consistency, and low in consensus.

Several investigators have reported evidence supporting Kelley's (1967) ideas. In a well-known study, McArthur (1972) examined the causal attributions made by observers of another person's behavior. She presented subjects with person–entity statements (e.g., "Tom is enthralled by the painting") and three accompanying statements providing information about high or low consensus (high: "Almost everyone who sees the painting is enthralled by it"), distinctiveness (high: "Tom is not enthralled by almost every other painting"), and consistency (high: "In the past, Tom has almost always been enthralled by the same painting"). For each set of information, the subjects were asked to decide what probably caused the event (e.g., Tom was enthralled by the painting) to occur. Subjects could attribute it to something about the person, something about the entity, something about the particular circumstance, or some combination of two or more of the first three factors. McArthur found that entity attribution (i.e., something about the painting) was relatively frequent when a response was characterized by high consensus, high distinctiveness, and high consistency. She also found that person attribution (i.e., something about Tom) was relatively frequent when a behavior was characterized by low consensus, low distinctiveness, and high consistency. In general, McArthur's results suggest that people can assimilate rather intricate combinations of information and make logical (in the manner suggested by Kelley) inferences based on that information.

Qualifying Research

While several investigators have replicated the main findings of McArthur (Ruble & Feldman, 1976; Zuckerman, 1978), there also has been some controversy regarding attributors' use of the three types of information specified by Kelley in his ANOVA model. Since much of the debate has focused on the role of consensus information in verifying whether causes and effects have been correctly linked, in this section we will review briefly the evidence relevant to this controversy.

The consensus debate really began with a set of studies in which Nisbett and Borgida (1975) found no evidence that consensus affects attributions. In one of these studies, they gave subjects a description of a study of helping behavior carried out by Darley and Latane (1968). After receiving the description, subjects were provided with the results of the study (the consensus information). For example, some were told that of 15 persons witnessing an epileptic seizure, 6 failed to do anything to help; other subjects were not given this information. Then subjects were told that one of the subjects, Greg R., never helped the person suffering the seizure. Subjects were asked to explain Greg R.'s behavior by indicating to what extent the situation or Greg R.'s personality had been the cause of his behavior. The consensus information was effective in the sense that the subjects receiving the information indicated that more participants in the study of helping never helped than did subjects in the no-information conditions. However, consensus had no effect on attributions about Greg R.'s behavior; subjects exhibited no significant differences in attributing Greg R.'s behavior to the situation or his personality. Based on reasoning from Kelley's (1967) analysis, it would have been expected that subjects would attribute Greg R.'s behavior more to the situation in the high-consensus (i.e., where six people never helped) condition than in the no-consensus-information condition. Nisbett and Borgida concluded that ". . . base rate information [such as consensus data] concerning categories in a population is *ignored* in estimating category membership of a sample of the population" (1975, p. 935) [our emphasis].

Subsequent research (Wells & Harvey, 1977) showed consensus effects under a stronger manipulation of consensus information and when it was stressed that the persons constituting the consensus sample were randomly selected. However, more recent work by Major (1980) revealed the weakness of consensus information relative to distinctiveness and consistency information in a situation in which subjects could ask for different types of information to explain why an event occurred. Also, Hansen and Donoghue (1977) provided evidence that attributions are more affected by knowledge of one's own behavior (self-based consensus) than by others' behavior (sample-based consensus). This finding, however, was disputed by Kulik and Taylor (1980), who found that both types of consensus affect trait attributions.

As the subsequent research suggests, the consensus-attribution controversy appears to be virtually resolved by the delineation of several conditions under which consensus is and is not influential. In a useful review, Kassin (1979) suggested that consensus effects depend upon such mediating factors as the strength of magnitude of the base rate information, the salience of the information and the ease with which it may be applied, the perceived representativeness (and hence generalizability of the base rate sample), and the causal relevance of the base rate. Kassin also distinguishes between implicit and explicit consensus. Implicit consensus refers to subjective—often normative—expectancies for behavior in a situation, while explicit consensus refers to the actual behavior of individuals in a sample. Kassin contends that the type of consensus and/or the discrepancy between types may be crucial to whether or not such information affects attribution. Another useful review of the current state of affairs with consensus effects is provided by Borgida and Brekke (1981).

Causal Schemata

Kelley (1972a) suggests that while the ANOVA model is appropriate for certain cases in which the individual can engage in a relatively complete causal analysis, it is not descriptive of most attributional work. According to Kelley, the inferential problem is only infrequently so imposing that it necessitates a full-blown analysis. In many situations, we do not have time to engage in a complete analysis, even if it were advisable. The requirements of modern life frequently lead to hasty deliberations in which decisions are made by reference mainly to present feelings, thoughts, and perceptions, the advice of others, and our past experience. Kelley contends that past experience may provide individuals with a backlog of understanding relative to causal relations and that individuals can call on this store of knowledge when an inference has to be made quickly. This store of knowledge of causal relations represents what Kelley refers to as *causal schemata*. Kelley says that causal schemata are learned, stored in the person's memory, and then activated by environmental cues. Schemata presumably generalize on the basis of a broad range of objects and situations, and may be stimulated by numerous cues.[1] The types of schemata specified in Kelley's analysis include an attributor's tendency to invoke multiple sufficient causes (either cause A or cause B suffices to produce the effect) and multiple necessary causes (both A and B are necessary for the effect).

Only a few studies have been conducted to test these causal schemata ideas. There are many unanswered questions relating to schemata. For example, how do they develop? Are there pronounced differences among people in their schemata or their use of them? What are the most meaningful schemata? In what situations are they typically activated? An initial answer to this latter question was provided by Cunningham and Kelley (1975). They showed that effects of moderate magnitude are interpreted according to a multiple sufficient cause schema, while effects of extreme magnitude are interpreted according to a multiple necessary cause schema. (We will return to a discussion of the attributional schema notion in chap. 3.)

Discounting

The idea of *discounting* in attribution was articulated by Kelley in another of his important statements (Kelley, 1972b). This principle relates to the situation involving an attributor who has information about a given effect(s) and a number of possible causes. How are certain causes dis-

---

[1] Although Heider does not label this backlog of past experience as schemata, he too seems to be advancing a notion similar to causal schemata in his assertion that people readily make hundreds of attributions every day.

counted and others regarded as the real cause? Kelley offers this definition for discounting: "The role of a given cause in producing a given effect is discounted if other plausible causes are also present" (1972b, p. 8). Kelley suggests that discounting is reflected in ways such as a person's feeling of little certainty in the inference that a particular cause led to a particular effect. For example, suppose a male tells a wealthy female that she is one of the most lovely females in the city; she may feel little certainty about the sincerity of the compliment if she assumes that the male may be trying to get some monetary benefit from interacting with her. (A similar point is made in a study reported by Sigall & Michela, 1976.)

A classic pair of investigations by Thibaut and Riecken (1955) illustrates quite well how the discounting principle works in attributional activity. In one of two parallel studies, an undergraduate male student worked with two other male subjects, who were both actually the experimenter's accomplices. One of the accomplices was revealed to be of higher status (he had just finished his PhD requirements) than the other subject, who presumably had just finished his freshman year of college. As the experimental procedure developed, the true subject found it necessary to attempt to influence the two accomplices to help him. Eventually, and at the same time, both agreed to do so. Compliance by the accomplices constituted the effect for which the subject had various plausible causal explanations. He was asked whether each person complied because he wanted to (an internal cause) or because he had been forced to (an external cause). The results showed that subjects attributed the high-status person's compliance to the internal cause and the low-status person's compliance to the external cause.

How does this study illustrate the discounting principle? The possible internal cause of compliance by both the high- and low-status persons is the person's own preference, and the external cause is the subject's persuasive power. In the case of the high-status person, the subject's power is not a plausible cause for compliance, and given the two plausible causes (including the low-status person's own preference), the role of the internal cause is discounted; thus, the low-status person's behavior is attributed to external pressure.[2]

Augmentation

When there are multiple plausible causes of a given effect and when some of these causes are facilitative and others are inhibitory with respect to the effect, a reverse version of the discounting principle, which has been called

---

[2]The astute reader may recognize the similarity between Kelley's discounting principle and Jones and Davis's (1965) noncommon-effect analysis. According to Jones and Davis, correspondence of inferences increases as the number of noncommon effects (in Kelley's terminology, the number of plausible causes) decreases.

the *augmentation principle*, is necessary. Kelley has defined this augmentation principle as follows: "If for a given effect, both a plausible inhibitory cause and a plausible facilitative cause are present, the role of the facilitative cause in producing the effect will be judged greater than if it alone were present as a plausible cause for the effect" (1972b, p. 12). The important idea in this definition is that the facilitative cause must have been extremely potent if the effect occurred despite the opposing effect of the inhibitory cause. For example, if we were to observe an individual perform extremely well on the Graduate Record Examination, despite the fact that this individual was obviously not feeling well, we would likely overattribute successful performance (in the face of plausible external reasons for unsuccessful performance) to the individual's ability or effort.

Kelley (1972b) reviews a large body of evidence that relates to the discounting and augmentation principles. In some of this research, it is hard to tell whether there is evidence of one or both principles. However, a study reported by Himmelfarb and Anderson (1975) provides clear evidence for both. Additionally, more recent research (Hansen & Hall, 1985) suggests that (a) discounting may be more potent than augmentation, and (b) the magnitude of a given effect produced by facilitative forces opposed by inhibitory forces has more impact on the perceived strength of the facilitative than on the perceived strength of the inhibitory forces. These findings suggest that attributors may overlook or have difficulty using information about negative as opposed to positive causation.

It seems likely that discounting and augmentation processes will continue to represent a focal topic for future research in attribution theory. Theoretically, there are a number of major questions that remain to be investigated, including: What decisional rules do people use in deciding which of seemingly equivalent causes to discount? Do people often discount or augment the importance of plausible causes in line with their self-interests, as opposed to mainly rational considerations?

Concluding Points

In his various writings (especially 1967, 1972a, 1972b, 1973), Kelley has produced some of the most elegant and elaborate analyses of attributional processes that exist to date. It is important to note that while Kelley based his analyses of the attribution process on the covariation principle, a number of studies have found that people sometimes are not able to assess accurately covariation information (see reviews by Alloy & Tabachnik, 1984; Crocker, 1981; Nisbett & Ross, 1980). However, as Ross and Fletcher (1985) have noted, "That people may sometimes be poor detectors of 'objective' covariation does not undermine the covariation principle. . . . The perception of variance underlies causal inference. The degree to which such perceptions accurately mirror objective reality is a separate issue" (p. 83).

In summary, Kelley has made a notable attempt to synthesize person perception (other attribution) and self-perception concepts, and he has developed formal models of how people deliberately analyze information and make inferences, as well as models of how they do this very quickly. As was true of the theoretical work of Jones and colleagues, Kelley's analyses have been limited in terms of explaining how powerful motives and emotions interact with logical–rational processes to produce attributional phenomena.

Kruglanski's Lay Epistemology

Before turning to a discussion of Bem's early foundation work relevant to attribution processes, it is important to discuss briefly theoretical work by Kruglanski and his colleagues on what they refer to as *lay epistemology*. Kruglanski, Hamel, Maides, and Schwartz (1978) claimed that their approach subsumes Kelley's (1967) ANOVA model. Kruglanski and his colleagues drew distinctions among the content, logic, and course of epistemic behavior and provided this general description of their focus: "The content of naive epistemology is the laymen's total set of concepts pertaining to the world of experience. The epistemic logic is the assessment criterion, the fulfillment of which yields a sense of valid knowledge. The course of lay inquiry is the sequence of cognitive operations intended to assess the possibility of significant new knowledge" (1978, p. 302).

More specifically, Kruglanski et al. argued that the ANOVA model is concerned with a subset of attributional categories (person, entity, circumstance), while the epistemological formulation permits evaluation of other potential categories of causes of events. These authors also contended that the ANOVA model concerns only one type of relation that may be of interest to attributors—causality; the epistemological formulation takes into consideration other types of relations (e.g., logical, spatial, temporal). Additionally, Kruglanski et al. argued that the logic underlying the ANOVA model (covariation) is a special case of a more general distinctiveness–consistency logic. Essentially, they argued that the lay attributor uses one type of logic in validating attributions, namely: The person considers a hypothesis such as "She is a kind person" by evaluating the consistency of the implications of the hypothesis. If they are consistent, the hypothesis is confirmed. For example, a person attribution (e.g., she is kind) requires *distinctiveness* (or covariation) between the specific person and an effect ("low consensus," in Kelley's terminology) and *consistency* across other plausible causes, for example, entity and circumstance ("time" and "modality").

The evidence Kruglanski et al. (1978) advanced to support their position is indirect and does not show that people necessarily feel that certain pieces of knowledge are consistent and others inconsistent. For example, they showed that people may have a relatively great preference for information that is highly relevant to an event (e.g., "John laughed at the comedian"); highly relevant information might include a means–ends datum such as, "The comedian is John's supervisor." The preference for this type of information is relative to general information believed to be important in other models (e.g., consensus, "Others did not laugh at the comedian").

These results help to illustrate the Kruglanski et al. position, but they do not show that people use only consistent criteria in making attributions. People cannot always calculate which information is consistent or highly relevant to an attribution. Also, in many situations there are mixes of data both consistent and inconsistent with early hypotheses we form. In these situations, the criteria described by theorists such as Heider, Kelley, and Jones are quite essential to the layperson. Clearly, an evaluation of the lay epistemology formulation awaits further and more direct empirical investigations.

Bem's Contribution to Attribution Theory

In this final section, we will review Daryl Bem's (1967a, 1972) seminal conceptions of how people interpret their own behavior and psychological states. The importance of Bem's contribution to the attribution area first was fully recognized by Kelley (1967) in his perceptive, integrative review. Kelley recognized Bem's work on self-perception as a necessary complement to the work by Jones and Davis and others on person perception. Bem (1972) has acknowledged and expanded on the attributional characteristics of his earlier work. This work now has become an important part of the attribution literature, even though it originally was intended to represent an alternative approach to dissonance theory in attitude change research.

Bem (1972) claims that people come to know their own attitudes, emotions, and other internal states partially by inferring them from observations of their own overt behavior and the context in which this behavior occurs. That is, people "look back" and imagine their acts together with the relevant situations in which they occurred, then infer their internal states by means of logical deduction (e.g., "If I was eating scallops, and no one was influencing me to eat them, then I must like scallops"). The strikingly unorthodox implication of Bem's analysis is that people do not know what they think, feel, or believe before they act. It follows, also, that Bem does not consider that attributional change occurs because people do not have prior attributions that exist apart from behavior. Rather, Bem asserted that people infer their internal states such as attributions and attitudes after they behave, and that they cannot remember internal states that are discrepant with their behavior (see Bem & McConnell, 1970). In this conception, people are viewed as strictly information processors, making attributions about themselves based mainly upon observable data. Bem's central proposition is: "Individuals come to 'know' their own attitudes, emotions, and other internal states partially by inferring them from observations of their own overt behavior and/or the circumstances in which this behavior occurs. Thus, to the extent that internal cues are weak, ambiguous, or uninterpretable, the individual is functionally in the same position as an outside observer who must necessarily rely upon those same external cues to infer the individual's inner states" (1972, p. 2).

Bem traces much of his work to Skinner's (1957) operant behavioristic analysis of human verbal behavior. Bem claims that his theory embodies radical behaviorism because it eschews any reference to internal physiological or conceptual processes. Bem's arguments have engendered considerable debate, especially in the attitude area (e.g., Bem, 1967b; Jones, Linder, Keisler, Zanna, & Brehm, 1968; Mills, 1967). However, his position has had considerable impact upon contemporary attribution work (e.g., Snyder, 1976). Bem (1972) contended that the 1960s had been dominated by theories concerned with chronic drives toward consistency and uncertainty reduction (e.g., dissonance theory), whereas the 1970s would be dominated by theories emphasizing rational contemplation and information processing. He argued that there was a paradigm shift occurring in social psychology, a shift from motivation/drive models of cognitions to information processing/attribution models—of which self-perception theory was an element. Bem was right, in part, and his theoretical work set the pace for this development, which will be discussed in greater length in chapters 2 and 3.

Concluding Points

Although Bem (1967a, 1967b, 1972) contended that his work embodied behaviorism, such a contention is not logically supported by the assumption that people infer their internal states. Further, Bem's central proposition, as quoted above, is full of theoretical loopholes—". . . to the extent that internal cues are weak, ambiguous, or uninterpretable. . . ." How do we know whether internal cues should be so characterized? Bem's statements are silent about such reservations as these. Bem's presumably nonmotivational perspective also does not address the question of why people make attributions. Indeed, to answer such a question would require invoking some motivational principle, such as a desire to understand or control one's social environment.

These points notwithstanding, Bem's influence has been important. His work has stimulated much research that is clearly attributional in character. Moreover, he was the first theorist concerned with attribution processes to focus exclusively upon self-perception and how people understand their personal states. Finally, Bem focused our attention on behavior to an extent few other contemporary theorists have; as Bem (1972) remarked, attributional analyses have been especially incomplete in treating the linkages among various types of overt behavior and various classes of cognitions/attributions, and also types of physiological responses.

A Brief Summary and Comparison of Basic Attribution Theories

Before moving on to a discussion of major theoretical qualifications, extensions, and advances, it may be helpful to point out briefly some of the major distinctions between the approaches discussed so far. Heider's naive analysis of action was the germinal work for later theoretical developments; all subsequent analyses contained elements of Heider's formulation. Heider did not provide much empirical foundation for his ideas. Jones and Davis presented the first empirically grounded attribution statement. These theorists were concerned primarily with person-perception processes, and their analysis focused solely on determinants of attributions to other people. In particular, Jones and Davis were concerned with how perceivers make attributions about the intentions and dispositions of other people. In contrast, Bem's work was concerned solely with the process of self-attribution. He theorized about the process whereby people find out about their own internal states, such as attitudes, beliefs, and emotions. Bem also provided an empirical foundation for much of his theorizing on self-perception processes. Kelley's early work was aimed at synthesizing and integrating work on self and other attributional processes. Recently, empirical investigations of his own particular versions of attribution theory have been actively pursued.

2
Theoretical Qualifications and Extensions

In this chapter, we will review theoretical qualifications and extensions in the attribution area that were prominent in the 1970s and early 1980s. Our treatment will be general and selective. We will describe a continuation of theoretical and empirical work based on the beginning foundation writings of Heider, Jones and colleagues, Kelley, and Bem. We will note how much of this continuation work has generated a good deal of research, debate, and, in some cases, clarification of basic process issues. But we also will point out how these theoretical qualifications and extensions of the 1970s, for the most part, have not led to the type of broad, systematic analyses of attributional phenomena that might have been expected in light of Heider's (1958) magnum opus and the rush of theoretical work in the mid- and late 1960s.

The topics to be covered in this chapter on qualifications and extensions are:

1. Measurement of attribution
2. Nature of attribution
3. Actor–observer differences in attributed causality
4. Motivational processes in attributional activities
5. Misattribution of arousal
6. A brief commentary on the significance of these qualifications and extensions

Measurement of Attribution

We already have documented the volume of production of research in the attribution area that has occurred over the last several decades. What is surprising, given this volume of work, is that until relatively recently little research has focused on the measurement of attributions and related theoretical issues.

Assessment of Causal Factors

In attribution studies, there are a number of methods that have been used to assess causal attributions. These include (a) open-ended measures (i.e., subjects list what they believe to be the cause or causes of an event, and then the coder classifies subjects' attributions as ability attributions, effort attributions, or other relevant categories of causal factors), (b) independent ratings (i.e., ratings of the importance of specified causes of the event), (c) percentage of causality measures in which the totality of percentages of possible, specified causes of the event must equal 100% (sometimes called ipsative measures because the assignment of a percentage to one cause of the event influences the percentage of contribution of other specified causes), (d) choice of one major cause, and (e) bipolar ratings (two possible causes of the event—ability and luck, for example—anchor the endpoints of the scale).

One major distinction among these measures is whether the potential causes for the event are specified on some a priori basis and presented by the experimenter or are generated by subjects. In the former instance, the fixed list of potential causes rated or selected by subjects generally is based on theoretical considerations. For example, based on Heider's (1958) distinction of causal factors internal and external to the person involved in the event, the experimenter may present subjects with a fixed list of internal factors such as ability and effort and external factors such as task difficulty and luck. A critical question, of course, is the degree to which ordinary people make such causal distinctions. Perhaps other causal factors such as the person's mood or other people are viewed as important by subjects (Elig & Frieze, 1975).

In perhaps the most comprehensive examination of measurement issues, Elig and Frieze (1979) evaluated three different methods of assessing causal attributions: open-ended responses, percentage ratings (equaling 100%), and independent ratings of importance. In this study, college students made attributions on all three measures for their success or failure on an anagram task. The measures then were evaluated in terms of how reliable (repeatable) and valid (whether they measured what they were supposed to measure) they were. Elig and Frieze concluded from their analyses that the independent rating measures were more reliable and valid than were the percentage or open-ended methods of assessing causal attributions. While they recommended use of the independent scales in settings where the potential causal factors are relatively well-understood (e.g., achievement settings), they also noted that open-ended measures may prove very useful when researchers are assessing causal attributions in novel situations.

Assessment of Causal Dimensions

An issue related to the measurement of specific causal factors is the adequacy of various measures of causal dimensions. Researchers often are more interested in assessing the dimensional characteristics (e.g., internal–external) underlying attributions than the specific causal attributions per se (e.g., ability or task difficulty), and they typically use one of two general procedures to identify the relevant dimensions. More specifically, researchers may translate specific attributions made by subjects into some dimensional categorization based on the theoretical meaning of the cause. For example, if a subject attributes his or her success on a class exam to high ability, the experimenter would classify this specific attribution as *internal* to the subject and as *stable*, or invariant over time (Weiner, 1972; see also chap. 9). This procedure, of course, assumes that the theoretical meaning attached to a specific cause by the experimenter is consistent with the meaning of the cause to the attributor. Alternatively, researchers may directly ask subjects for their perceptions of the causes.

In a recent study, Russell, McAuley, and Tarico (1987) compared the relability and validity of three different measures of attributional dimensions. In a manner similar to Elig and Frieze (1979), Russell et al. asked subjects, following receipt of an exam grade, to make attributions for their performance. The dimensions underlying these attributions were assessed in three different ways. First, subjects were asked to indicate on the Causal Dimension Scale (Russell, 1982) their perceptions of the causes of their exam performance in terms of the locus of causality (internal–external), stability, and controllability dimensions identified in previous research to be important in achievement-related settings. Second, subject's attributions were coded by judges along the three attributional dimensions.

The third method of determining dimensional ratings entailed asking subjects to rate the importance of a number of specified potential causal factors to their exam performance. These factors were classified on theoretical grounds as representing one end of the three dimensions of locus of causality, stability, and controllability. A difference score of the sum of ratings of causes at one end of a continuum was subtracted from the sum of ratings at the other end. For example, the importance ratings for task difficulty and luck (external factors) were subtracted from the ratings of ability and effort (internal factors). The resulting score indicated the relative importance of causes along an internal–external locus of causality dimension.

The results of this study provided support for directly assessing how subjects perceive the causes they cite for their achievement outcome. While both the open-ended measure and the Causal Dimension Scale proved to be reliable methods of assessing causal dimensions, the Causal Dimension Scale was more valid than either of the other measures. An additional finding of this study was that across all three methods of assessment, the locus of causality and controllability dimensions were highly intercorrelated. It may be that in some situations these two dimensions are naturally related, while the causal structure of other situations may produce an independence of them (see also Anderson & Arnoult, 1985).

In another investigation of methods of assessing causal dimensions, Solomon (1978) examined three commonly used measurement techniques employing importance ratings. He argued that researchers have been assuming an inverse relationship between internal (dispositional) and external (situational) dimensions of attributions (i.e., as the perceived importance of one increases, the importance of the other decreases) when they ask subjects to rate on a bipolar scale the relative importance of such factors, or when they combine subjects' ratings on two scales by subtracting the external rating from the internal rating. The results of Solomon's comparison of bipolar, combined ratings and ratings made on independent scales indicate that internal and external attributions are not inversely related and may vary along different dimensions. Consequently, only studies that report internal and external attributions separately allow us to draw unambiguous conclusions.

Concluding Points

Kelley and Michela (1980) have noted that ". . . the central irony of attribution research is that while its central concepts concern the causal distinctions made by common people, these have been little investigated" (p. 490). From the brief review of research presented above, we can see that some progress has been made both in terms of understanding the specific attributions made by ordinary people as well as their perceptions of the relevant underlying causal dimensions. Progress also has been made in terms of the measurement of specific attributions and the causal dimensions underlying them. It is important to note, however, that both of the major comparisons of measures discussed above (Elig & Frieze, 1979; Russell, McAuley, & Tarico, 1987) focused on a single setting; that is, both studies examined attributions for achievement outcomes. Other studies (Anderson, 1983a; Russell et al., 1985; Wimer & Kelley, 1982) have examined attributions in a wide variety of settings and have found that causal attributions and dimensions can vary considerably from situation to situation. Indeed, it appears that "people can make whatever distinctions their language permits and the causal structures of their world make important" (Wimer & Kelley, 1982, p. 1161). Clearly, future research applying attribution conceptions to novel situations may need to be concerned with a situation-specific determination of the relevant causal factors and dimensions.

Nature of Attribution

During the past decade, considerable debate has occurred regarding the nature of attributions. A number of diverse topics have been addressed in the literature. In this section, we will review the debate surrounding questions about the extent to which attributions are accurate or inaccurate, whether they are represented in statements of reasons as well as statements of causes, and the impact of cultural meaning systems on the development of causal inferences.

Accuracy of Attributions

As we noted in chapter 1, the major goal of attributional processes is to render the social world understandable, predictable, and controllable. It therefore should surprise no one that the degree of accuracy of our attributions has been a topic of some considerable interest and controversy. While a number of potential biases, or errors, in attributions have been investigated, perhaps the best-documented one is the so-called "fundamental attribution error" (Ross, 1977), or "overattribution effect" (Jones, 1979). Both of these terms refer to the pervasive tendency of attributors ". . . to overestimate the importance of personal or dispositional factors relative to environmental influences" (Ross, 1977, p. 184).

Attributors' inclination to overattribute to dispositional factors has long been recognized as a prominent attributional tendency (Heider, 1958) and has received support primarily from research employing the attitude-attribution paradigm. In a classic study, Jones and Harris (1967) presented subjects with pro- or anti-Castro essays purportedly written by a target person who had no choice in what to write (low-choice conditions) or freely chose the essay position (high-choice conditions). Subjects' task was to infer the true attitude of the essay writer. Consistent with correspondent inference theory (Jones & Davis, 1965), subjects in the Jones and Harris (1967) study attributed stronger essay-consistent attitudes in the high-choice than in the low-choice conditions. However, even in the low-choice conditions they still attibuted relatively correspondent attitudes to the essay writer.

This tendency to overattribute to the target and to discount to too great a degree the situational constraints on the target's behavior has been demonstrated in a wide variety of contexts and generally has been viewed as a serious judgmental error. Despite the robustness of the overattribution effect, considerable controversy remains about at least two issues: Does it represent a fundamental error in human judgmental processes, and how should the effect be interpreted? Let us take each of these questions in turn.

A number of investigators have questioned whether the overattribution effect represents a judgmental error (Funder, 1982, Hamilton, 1980; Harvey, Town, & Yarkin, 1981). Among the issues raised are: (a) what criteria to use in establishing the accuracy of attribution (Harvey et al., 1981); (b) whether under certain conditions an overattribution to situational factors may occur and may also represent an "error." In this regard, Quattrone (1982) has shown that using a procedure similar to that employed in the typical attitude-attribution study, subjects can be led to overattribute to the situation if the experimenter just asks them to use the essay to estimate the situational forces that might be present, rather than the essay writer's true attitude; and (c) the idea that an important difference between situational and dispositional attributions is the level of analysis. That is, situational attributions describe environmental circumstances associated with behavior, while dispositional attributions are intended to describe how a given action fits into the larger pattern of the actor's behavior over time (Funder, 1982).

In surely the most comprehensive treatment to date of issues surrounding the issue of the accuracy of social judgments, Funder (1987) has distinguished between "errors" and "mistakes" in inferential processes.

An "error" is a judgment of a laboratory stimulus that deviates from a model of how that judgment should be made. . . . A "mistake," by contrast, is an incorrect judgment in the real world . . . and so must be determined by different criteria. Detection of an error implies the existence of a mistake *only* when the process that produces the error also produces incorrect judgment in real life. Unfortunately, this cannot be determined by merely demonstrating the error itself, because the same judgment that is wrong in relation to a laboratory stimulus, taken literally, may be right in terms of a wider, more broadly defined social context, and reflect processes that lead to accurate judgments under ordinary circumstances (p. 76).

In terms of the attitude-attribution paradigm, Funder argues that subjects' responses to the wider social context of the experimental procedure make perfect sense. It is not surprising that subjects make the "error" of basing their inferences about the essay writer's attitude on the information they have been given (the essay content), and this "error" should not be viewed as a "mistake." For the overattribution effect to be seen as a mistake would require researchers to let subjects judge real people in authentic social situations and to use realistic, external criteria for assessing when these judgments are accurate or inaccurate.

Whatever the ultimate resolution of issues about error, there is little controversy about the empirical status of the overattribution effect. As we noted earlier, it is a very robust finding. Exactly how to interpret the effect is, however, another matter. A recent study by Tetlock (1985) sheds some light on this question. Tetlock reasoned that if subjects were motivated to process carefully the information provided by the experimenter, then the overattribution to the essay writer's dispositional characteristics might not occur. To test this hypothesis, he had subjects read pro- or anti-affirmative-action essays that were written under low- or high-choice conditions. In addition, he led some subjects to believe that they would have to justify their impressions of the essay writer. The results indicated that when subjects did not feel accountable for their impressions, evidence of the usual overattribution effect was obtained. Subjects, however, were considerably more sensitive to the situational causes of the essay writer's behavior when, prior to receiving the stimulus information, they felt accountable for their impressions.

The results of Tetlock's (1985) study shed some light not only on cognitive processes underlying the overattribution effect, but perhaps also on those underlying other cognitive biases. They also suggest that there may be a relatively effective social strategy for "de-biasing" or checking cognitive processes that result in "erroneous" judgments.

Causes and Reasons, Endogenous and Exogenous Behavior

Several theorists have argued that the theoretical distinctions made by early writers of the various causal dimensions (internal–external, stable–unstable, controllable–uncontrollable) were overly simplistic and have resulted in no small amount of conceptual confusion in the literature. Two potentially useful distinctions that have more recently been proposed are: (a) Buss's (1978) argument that "causes" represent the necessary and sufficient conditions for a behavior and that "reasons" represent the purposes or goals of a behavior; and (b) Kruglanski's (1975, 1979) distinction between explanations of behavior as "endogenous" (the behavior as an end in itself) versus "exogenous" (the behavior as a means to a further end). This latter distinction was offered as a replacement for the internal–external partition that has been used so extensively in attribution research. While both Buss and Kruglanski at least imply that people are aware of such distinctions in their attributional activities, there is little evidence one way or another on this possibility. Indeed, despite a modicum of empirical work on the endogenous–exogenous distinction—much of which has been carried out by Kruglanski and his colleagues—as well as several attempts to clarify conceptual difficulties surrounding Buss's cause–reason distinction (Harvey & Tucker, 1979; Kruglanski, 1979; Locke & Pennington, 1982) and several studies by Zuckerman and his colleagues (Zuckerman & Evans, 1984; Zuckerman & Feldman, 1984) suggesting that voluntary behaviors (actions) are likely to be interpreted in terms of reasons whereas involuntary ones (occurrences) are likely to be interpreted in terms of causes, little systematic attention has been given to them among attribution researchers. The distinctions made in earlier foundation work continue to be more widely used, perhaps because of their intuitive appeal and appearance as constructs in attributors' everyday language and thinking (cf. Schoeneman & Rubanowitz, 1985).

Cultural Meaning Systems and Attributions

One theme that has been present in our discussions of measurement issues and theoretical distinctions of attributions is the notion that the specific attributional content used by people can vary from situation to situation. To this we must add the probably obvious point that attributional content also may vary from one culture to another. That diversity in language and associated cultural meaning systems can influence the causal inference process, while perhaps obvious, has not been the focus of widespread empirical inquiry. A notable exception is a recent study (Miller, 1984) of the impact of Western (U.S.) and non-Western (India) cultural conceptions on attributional processes.

The possibility of situational and cultural diversity in attributional contents raises some troublesome concerns for attribution theorists and researchers. After all, the goal of scientific psychology is to develop universal principles, and "preoccupation with [numerous] lay concepts threatens to ensnare attribution theory in endless particularities that might ultimately divest it of scientific value" (Kruglanski, 1979, p. 1447). At least one theorist, however, has suggested a possible solution to this potential, undesirable state of affairs. Specifically, Kruglanski et al. (1978) have suggested that while attributional *contents* might be specific to situations and cultures, the logic (Kelley's covariation principle and Kruglanski's consistency principle, see chap. 1) used to validate specific attributions is universal and invariant. Moreover, Kruglanski (1979) has argued that theory should be concerned with this universal logic, or process, underlying knowledge acquisition, not the diverse contents of such social knowledge. While the distinction between specific attributional contents and a universal logic is interesting, the assertion that the latter is universal across cultures and situations surely will need empirical investigation.

Actor–Observer Differences in Attributed Causality

Jones and Nisbett's Divergent Perspectives Hypothesis

One of the provocative extensions of basic attribution ideas has been concerned with the question of how people with different perspectives diverge in their attributions about the causes of the same behavior. This concern with divergence in attribution emanates mainly from Jones and Nisbett's (1972) influential theoretical statement on actor–observer differences in the attribution of causality. Jones and Nisbett's analysis was influenced in part by the following ideas presented by Heider (1958): "It seems that behavior in particular has such salient properties it tends to engulf the total field rather than be confined to its proper position as local stimulus whose interpretation requires the additional data of a surrounding field—the situation in social perception" (p. 54); and "The person tends to attribute his own reactions to the object world, and those of another, when they differ from his own to personal characteristics in O [other]" (p. 157).

In their statement, Jones and Nisbett (1972) hypothesize that actors will attribute causality or responsibility for their behavior to situational influences, whereas observers will attribute causality for the same behavior to stable dispositions possessed by the actors. Jones and Nisbett argue that actors and observers frequently possess different background data for evaluating the significance of an action. Actors generally know more about their behavior and present experiences than do observers. Jones and Nisbett suggest that this background knowledge may divert actors from making a dispositional attribution; that is, actors' attributions may be influenced by their recollection that their behavior has shown variance in similar situations in the past. Observers probably lack information about the distinctiveness and consistency of the actors' behavior. Because of this deficiency in background data, observers may tend to focus their causal analysis on actors and their presumed stable personality dispositions.

As an example of how this actor–observer bias might operate in a natural setting, consider a situation in which a medium-sized city has been in great financial distress for many years, but then after a new city manager takes office, the city's situation improves to the point of much economic prosperity and promise. The city's residents, not having a full understanding of the influences on the city's economy, may attribute the prosperity to the new manager's ability. The city manager, however, may attribute the emerging prosperity to the correction of past mismanagement of city funds, help from the federal government, and a new tax on items commonly bought by tourists visiting the city—all external situational–circumstantial factors.

Jones and Nisbett also contend that different aspects of the available information are salient for actors and observers, and that this differential salience affects the course and outcome of the attribution process. Because actors' sensory receptors are poorly located for observing themselves in action, they may tend to direct their attention to the situational cues with which their behavior is coordinated. To actors, these salient aspects of the environment are the determinants of their behavior. From the observer's perspective, these situational cues may be obscured by the actors' behavior (Heider's "behavior engulfs the field" idea; see also Taylor & Fiske, 1978). The observer, therefore, may tend to assign major responsibility for the actors' behavior to dispositional qualities possessed by the actors.

Evidence About Actor–Observer Attributional Difference

Nisbett, Caputo, Legant, and Maracek (1973) and Storms (1973) provided early evidence relevant to Jones and Nisbett's divergent perspectives hypothesis. Nisbett and associates created one experimental situation in which observers watched actors either comply with or refuse an experimenter's request that they volunteer their time in service on a particular project for their university. As the investigators had predicted, observers tended to assume that actors would behave in the future in ways similar to those they had just witnessed, whereas actors made no inferences about their own future behavior. In other words, observers saw actors as very fixed and static in their behavior, but actors did not have the same image of themselves. Actors perhaps thought that their future behavior would depend on the circumstances prevailing at that time. In a second study by Nisbett et al. (1973) indirect support for the divergent perspectives hypothesis was revealed in the finding that college students described their best friends' choice of girl friends and college majors by reference to the dispositional qualities of their best friends but they described their own similar choice in terms of the properties of the girl friends or majors.

Storms (1973) provided more direct evidence that an observer attributes an actor's behavior to his or her disposition, whereas the actor attributes the same behavior to the situation. Storms used videotape to provide the actors with a repeated view of their original visual orientations or with a new view of the observer's visual orientation of the actors' behavior (a simple disucssion between two people); the observers received either a repeated view of actors or a new visual orientation of how actors saw the situation. Importantly, Storms showed that the actor–observer tendency hypothesized by Jones and Nisbett can be observed if actors and observers maintain their usual visual perspective but that, with a reversal of perspective, the tendency can be reversed, the observer now making more situational attributions than the actor.

Storms's study provides evidence in support of Jones and Nisbett's (1972) argument that actor–observer divergencies are due in part to differential foci of attention; his results suggest that when the foci are reversed, the attributional divergencies may be reversed too. More recent evidence suggests that reversing the informational rather than the visual perspective available to actors and observers also reverses attributional divergencies (Eisen, 1979).

Some Qualifying Evidence

Harvey, Arkin, Gleason, and Johnston (1974) and Harvey, Harris, and Barnes (1975) have found that observers are sensitive to the conditions surrounding an actor's behavior and do not simply make attributions to the actor without consideration of those conditions. Jones and Nisbett's (1972) statement does not include how contextual conditions might affect an observer's attributions to an actor. In the study by Harvey et al. (1974), actors took actions that were expected to have and actually did have either a positive or a negative outcome. When the effect was *discrepant* with the expectation (for example, when a positive outcome had been expected, but a negative outcome occurred), observers who were in the same situation attributed much more causality to the actor than they did when the effect was not discrepant. Harvey and associates argued that a discrepancy between expected and actual events makes the actor's behavior highly salient and hence draws observers' attributions to him or her.

In the study by Harvey et al. (1975), actors took actions that had either a moderately negative or a strongly negative effect on another person. The results showed that the actors attributed less responsibility to themselves the more negative the effect on the other person. The authors argued that these results reflected actors' need to maintain self-esteem in light of a potentially culpable personal act. It also was found that the more negative the effect, the more responsibility the observers attributed to the actor. Presumably, according to Harvey et al. (1975), observers feel a greater need to control the actor's behavior the more negative it is, and they use their attributions toward attainment of this goal.

Additional support for this motivational interpretation of actor–observer attributional differences for positive and negative behaviors has been offered by Eisen (1979). Recall that one explanation offered by Jones and Nisbett for actor– observer attributional differences is that they have different information available to them. The actor presumably "knows" that his or her behavior has varied across situations, while the observer, not having such knowledge, may assume more behavioral consistency on the part of the actor. Eisen's (1979) findings supported Jones and Nisbett's notion that actors and observers make different assumptions about the consistency and distinctiveness of a given behavior. However, the results of this study suggested that such differences were due not so much to differential information, but were determined more by motivational factors (the desirability of the behavior). That is, negative behaviors were seen as more distinctive whereas positive behaviors were seen as more consistent by actors than observers.

A Methodological Note

Since the publication of Jones and Nisbett's (1972) statement, considerable work has been directed toward examining conditions under which *qualifications* of the divergent perspectives tendency will obtain. Much of this work is reviewed by Zuckerman (1979). A conclusion emerging from this review is that while many qualifying conditions have been specified, comparison of the results of studies is difficult because of the diversity of procedures used. For example, in some studies, subjects play the role of actors or observers in hypothetical situations, whereas, in other studies, actors and observers are present in either interpersonal-influence or achievement–performance situations. Significantly, it may be concluded from Zuckerman's review that quite different results may be expected for the same variables in these different research settings. The import of this conclusion is revealed most clearly by consideration of the paradigm in which people are asked to imagine being actors or observers in a hypothetical situation. These subjects are not apt to experience the level of involvement felt by actual actors and observers. Consequently, their attributional tendencies may be relatively tempered. Hypothetical actors may experience little of the motivational tension that may occur often when success or failure or positive or negative outcomes are associated with behavior. Furthermore, hypothetical observers do not have the literal focus on an actor and the actor's behavior—a focus which may intensify dispositional attributional tendencies. Logically, there are so many differences between hypothetical and participant situations that it is virtually impossible to assess clearly the comparability of operations and data.

Although the hypothetical situation format was useful in early work in various areas of attribution research, it seems clear that future work will have a stronger potential for ecological generalizability to the extent that more involving situations are sampled (Cutrona, Russell, & Jones, 1985; Hammen & Cochran, 1981; Miller, Klee, & Norman, 1982). Also, a concerted focus on such situations may lead to more coherence in findings and qualifying conclusions relevant to the divergent perspectives hypothesis.

Reformulation

In a step toward reformulating the divergent perspectives hypothesis, Monson and Snyder (1977) reviewed data relevant to this hypothesis and developed a number of qualifying propositions. Based upon their assessment of the evidence, Monson and Snyder suggested that when a behavior has been performed in a situation *chosen* by the actor, actors will make more dispositional attributions than will observers. However, they also suggested that for behaviors performed in situations not chosen by the actor, actors will make more situational attributions than will observers. Monson and Snyder further contended that, whether actors or observers, individuals may differ in a *general way* in their inclinations to make situational or dispositional inferences; some may be more inclined to be internal or external in a relatively pervasive way. (Recent support for such a general tendency has been reported by Fletcher, Danilovics, Fernandez, Peterson, & Reeder, 1986.) Monson and Snyder proposed that an actor's intentionality is a critical determinant of actor–observer differences. They contended that when an act leads to an outcome that is *not intended*, the attributions of actors ought to be more situational than those of observers. What about variables that specifically influence the observer? Monson and Snyder reviewed data showing that when observers are led to empathize with the actors' position, observers should be no more likely to make dispositional attributions than actors (Regan & Totten, 1975). This empathy-set variable is similar in its effect to the perspective-alteration variable examined by Storms (1973).

A study by Gould and Sigall (1977) provides further evidence about the role of empathy in influencing an observer's attributional perspective to become the functional equivalent of an actor's perspective. These investigators gave observers a set to empathize with a target person (e.g., observers were told, "While you are watching him, picture to yourself just how he feels. . . . Try to forget yourself"), or simply to observe the person. Subsequently, observers watched a videotape of a target male attempting to make a good first impression on a female. They then learned that the target person had either succeeded or failed at making a good first impression and were asked to make attributions for his outcome. As Gould and Sigall had predicted, observers given empathic instructions attributed the target person's success to dispositional causes and his failure to situational causes. That is, they exhibited a pattern generally similar to that shown by actors in research such as that by Harvey et al. (1974). Gould and Sigall's study provides further evidence about the importance of the interaction of the attributor's perspective (or cognitive set toward the event persons involved in it) and the nature or valence (e.g., positive or negative outcome) of the event in affecting how actors and observers will diverge or converge in their causal attributions.

Concluding Points About Actor–Observer Differences

Monson and Snyder concluded their analysis with the very reasonable suggestion that researchers turn from attempts to verify the divergent perspectives hypothesis to systematic investigations of the *when*, *why*, and *with what implications* for attribution theory of differences between actors and observers. A similar point was made by Watson (1982) in his review of the literature. Watson also concluded that while there is substantial evidence of the Target (actor vs. observer) × Type of Attribution (dispositional vs. situational) interaction predicted by Jones and Nisbett (1972), this interaction is due largely to the differential tendency of actors and observers to attribute causality to the environment, rather than to a differential preference for trait attributions; that is, both actors and observers consistently attribute more causal importance to dispositions than to situations.

Divergence in attribution would seem to represent an area that has major significance in many practical relationships (e.g., manager and worker, husband and wife, parent and child) and should continue to be a major area for attribution research in coming years. Indeed, research on actor–observer attributional divergencies has been influential in theoretical and empirical work concerned with attribution processes in close relationships (see chap. 5). Extensive knowledge of divergence is far from complete. For example, we know that people often take account of the persons with whom they will communicate their attributions and that this factor may influence actor–observer differences (see Wells, Petty, Harkins, Kagehiro, & Harvey, 1977). We also know that active observers' (those on the receiving end of the actor's behavior) attributions are more likely to be affected than passive observers' (onlookers of an event involving an actor and an observer) by the hedonic relevance and personalism of the actor's behavior (Cunningham, Starr, & Kanouse, 1979; Gilbert, Jones, & Pelham, 1987; Miller & Norman, 1975). However, we know little about the effects of different types of perceived social audiences or the various implications of the actor's behavior for different types of observers on actor–observer differences. We also know little about the impact of personality differences associated with actor–observer attributional asymmetries (Watson, 1982). As observed by Bem (1972), the full exploration of the rich and intriguing implications of Jones and Nisbett's divergent perspectives hypothesis will probably constitute a major direction in research on attributional processes for many years.

Motivational Processes in Attributional Activities

Investigations of attributional biases, such as the actor–observer differences proposed by Jones and Nisbett (1972) or the overattribution effect discussed by Ross (1977) and others, are of importance primarily because such biases may help us to elucidate basic attributional processes. Attribution theorists historically have been concerned with cognitive processes involved in self- and interpersonal perception, and perhaps for this reason most writers interested in attributional activities have stressed the importance of informational as opposed to motivational sources of bias (e.g., Bem, 1972; Jones & Nisbett, 1972; Kelley, 1967). This information-processing approach to understanding attributional biases has aroused considerable sympathy. Indeed, Ross (1977) has advocated that we abandon motivational concerns and concentrate on informational, perceptual, and cognitive factors that may account for systematic biases in attributions of causality. Other writers, however, have urged a more balanced approach in investigating potential mediating causes of attributional biases, noting that the most reasonable theory of the causal inference process likely will involve a precise articulation of the interaction of motivation and cognition (e.g., Shaver, 1975; Weary, 1980; Weary Bradley, 1978). In his seminal analyses of person perception and attribution processes, Heider also noted the necessity of considering the interdependence of motivation and cognition in attributional processes:

Since one's idea includes what "ought to be" and "what one would like to be" as well as "what is," attributions and cognitions are influenced by the mere subjective forces of needs and wishes as well as by the more objective evidence presented in the raw material (Heider, 1958, pp. 120–121).

In this section, we will examine research that focuses on the influence of two such "subjective forces": self-esteem and self-presentation.

Self-esteem

One of the more robust findings in social psychology is the tendency for individuals to accept more causal responsibility for their positive outcomes than for their negative outcomes (Greenwald, 1980; Weary Bradley, 1978). The operation of self-serving, or ego-defensive, biases has generally been used to explain these results. That is, by taking credit for good acts and denying blame for bad outcomes, an individual presumably is able to enhance or protect his or her self-esteem.

Miller and Ross (1975) questioned this motivational interpretation, suggesting that the results of many of the studies often cited as support for self-serving attributional biases could readily be "interpreted in information-processing terms' (p. 224). Specifically, these authors contended that the observed tendency for individuals to accept greater responsibility for positive than for negative outcomes may occur for any or all of several reasons: (a) individuals intend and expect success more than failure and are more likely to make self-ascriptions for expected than for unexpected outcomes; (b) perceived covariation between response and outcome may be more apparent for individuals experiencing a pattern of increasing success than for individuals experiencing constant failure; and (c) people erroneously base their judgments of the contingency between response and outcome on the occurrence of the desired outcome than on any actual degree of contingency.

Miller and Ross (1975) concluded that motivated distortions in the causal inference process had not been demonstrated. Kelley and Michela (1980) have argued, however, that more recent, methodologically improved studies of self-serving attributions are difficult to reinterpret in nonmotivational terms and consequently provide a fairly strong case for motivational effects (see reviews by Snyder, Stephan, & Rosenfield, 1978; Weary Bradley, 1978; Zuckerman, 1979). Indeed, since Kelley and Michela's (1980) review, a number of studies have investigated explicitly the presumed motivational mediators of self-serving attributional biases (e.g., Cohen, Dowling, Bishop, & Maney, 1985; McFarland & Ross, 1982; Stephan & Gollwitzer, 1981).

Weary (Weary, 1980; Weary Bradley, 1978) proposed that positive and negative affective states produced by success and failure experiences, respectively, mediate individuals' causal attributions for their behavioral outcomes. Specifically, she argued that self-enhancing attributions (i.e., high self-attributions) for success are mediated by and serve to maintain relatively high levels of positive affect, and self-protective attributions (i.e., low self-attributions following failure) are mediated by and function to alleviate high levels of negative affect (i.e., that self-protective attributions serve a threat-reducing purpose).

Gollwitzer, Earle, and Stephan (1982) designed a study to test this notion that outcome-related affect determines asymmetrical attributions for success and failure. In their study, Gollwitzer et al. used a technique based on excitation transfer theory (Zillmann, 1983) that permitted affect to be manipulated directly. Zillmann has suggested that the excitatory activity of emotions (positive and negative) is largely nonspecific and redundant. Therefore, residues of excitation from arousing tasks (e.g., physical exercise) can combine with and intensify subsequent affective states arising from a totally independent source. Gollwitzer et al. reasoned that outcome-related affect and self-serving biases would be exaggerated if performance feedback were given under conditions in which residues of excitation from prior stimulation combine with the excitatory reaction to performance feedback.

In their study, Gollwizer et al. had college students engage in physical exercise after working on a social perceptivity task. The students then were given success or failure feedback on the test either 1, 5, or 9 minutes after exercising. The results of this study indicated that self-serving attributional biases were exaggerated under conditions permitting the transfer of excitation from an irrelevant source. When students were highly aroused but could associate their arousal with the physical exercise (1-minute condition) or when their arousal produced by the exercise had dissipated (9-minute condition), their attributions for their outcomes on the social perceptiveness test were less self-serving than when residual arousal could be transferred to outcome-related affect (5-minute condition). It is difficult to see how these results could be explained in nonmotivational terms since the information processing interpretations of asymmetrical attributions for success and failure (Miller & Ross, 1975; Tetlock & Levi, 1982) assign no role to affect and arousal.

Other recent work on self-serving attributional biases has taken two general forms. First, researchers have attempted to establish boundary conditions for the positive–negative outcome attributional differences. For example, research on sex differences in attributions for one's own success or failure indicates that males exhibit the typical self-serving bias when the task is described as stereotypically masculine, while females show the usual positive–negative outcomes bias when the task is described as stereotypically feminine (Mirels, 1980; Rosenfield & Stephan, 1978). Individuals also exhibit the bias when their performance outcomes and attributions are private (Greenberg, Pyszczynski, & Solomon, 1982; Weary et al., 1982). Second, the generalizability of laboratory-based studies demonstrating self-serving biases to real-world settings has been a focus of research efforts. Investigators have found evidence of self-esteem biases in coaches' and players' attributions for their wins and losses (Carver, DeGregorio, & Gillis, 1980; Lau & Russell, 1980; Peterson, 1980) and in successful and unsuccessful medical school applicants' attributions for their admission decisions (Smith & Manard, 1980).

Approximately a decade ago, Weary argued that an important future task for researchers would seem to be uncovering ". . . how and under what conditions self-serving motivations influence attributions of causality" (Weary, 1979, p. 1419). As we pointed out above, researchers have made considerable progress in uncovering the "under what conditions" (i.e., the boundary conditions) of self-serving biases; they have been less focused in their attempts to elucidate the "how" or the precise process by which motivation influences the causal inference process. Such process issues can be expected to be a major and profitable direction of future research on motivational distortions in attributional processes.

Self-presentation

Within the last several years, attribution theorists and researchers have begun to recognize the possibility that individuals may express causal judgments that are designed to gain approval from or otherwise control the responses of others. For example, Weary (Weary, 1979; Weary Bradley, 1978) has contended that individuals may ascribe causality for positive and negative outcomes associated with their behaviors in such a way that would avoid embarrassment and/or gain public approval.

In testing for the operation of self-presentational motivations, investigators generally have employed two procedures: first, they have compared subjects' attributions under two conditions that are identical except that one is relatively private and the other is relatively public (e.g., Greenberg et al., 1982; Weary, 1980; Weary et al., 1982); and second, they have used the bogus pipeline (a bogus lie-detector apparatus) technique (Jones & Sigall, 1971) as a strategy for reducing distortion and dissimulation in verbal responses (e.g., Arkin, Appelman, & Burger, 1980; Riess, Rosenfeld, Melburg, & Tedeschi, 1981). If public awareness or potential discovery of misrepresentation affects attributors' communicated causal judgments, it presumably is because of their desire to create a favorable impression on others.

In one study, for example, Arkin et al. (1980) tested the notion, based on a self-presentation formulation, that individuals would become more modest about their abilities and attributes when others are not likely to be persuaded by or to challenge publicly a too positive interpretation of events. They found that participants accepted more credit for success than for failure when they did not expect their behavior to be evaluated by a group of experts. However, there was a reversal of this typical self-serving attributional bias among participants who were high in social anxiety and who expected their behavior to come under expert scrutiny. In a second experiment, this tendency for high-social-anxiety participants to accept more credit for failure than for success was replicated. Moreover, it was found that both high- and low-social-anxiety participants portrayed the causes of their performance outcomes in a more modest fashion when they responded via the bogus pipeline.

Arkin et al.'s (1980) results, then, support the premise that self-presentation motivations may bias causal attributions. They also shed some light on factors such as individual differences in social anxiety that may influence the choice of self-presentational strategy (e.g., modesty or self-enhancement). Other factors may include a variety of social-contextual factors prominently including the prestige of the audience. Indeed, research suggests that public evaluation of a person's performance by a committee of prestigious individuals leads to a moderation or reversal of self-enhancing attributional tendencies (e.g., Arkin et al., 1980; Greenberg et al., 1982), while observation of a person's performance by peers leads to an exaggeration of self-enhancing (or -protecting) causal attributions (Weary, 1980). A taxonomy of variables that may determine the precise influence of self-presentation motivations on attributors' causal judgments has been presented by Weary and Arkin (1981).

Considerable progress has been made in recognizing and understanding the role of self-presentation motives in attributional activities. Future directions for research may very well include examination of factors that determine the choice of a specific attributional self-presentation (see also chap. 7) and the effects of these strategies on audience reactions (Forsyth, Berger, & Mitchell, 1981; Tetlock, 1980) and on attributors' self-concepts.

Misattribution of Arousal

The one other extension of early theorizing to be described in this chapter concerns Zillmann's (1978) three-factor model of attribution of emotion. This model will be reviewed not because of its centrality as an attribution conception, but because of its extension of a very influential early work by Schachter and Singer (1962) concerned with the determinants of emotion (see also chap. 8 for a discussion of Schachter and Singer's work). Schachter and Singer's work deserves major attention because of its influence on attribution research. It has inspired theoretical and empirical work, controversy, and alternative models, such as Zillmann's conception. Interested readers should see Valins and Nisbett (1972) for further discussion of the stimulus value of Schachter and Singer's approach in attributional analyses.

Schachter and Singer's Work

Schachter and Singer (1962) proposed that cognitive factors and physiological arousal interact to produce emotion. They presented three main hypotheses:

1. Given a state of physiological arousal for which an individual has no immediate explanation, the individual will label this state and describe personal feelings in terms of available cognitions.

2. Given a state of physiological arousal for which an individual has a completely appropriate explanation, no evaluative needs will arise, and the individual is unlikely to label personal feelings in terms of available cognitions.
3. Given the same cognitive circumstances, the individual will react or describe personal feelings as emotions only to the extent that the individual experiences a state of physiological arousal.

Schachter and Singer's theoretical position is referred to as a two-factor model because of its emphasis upon physiological arousal and interpretation. In this account, heightened, diffuse arousal requires an explanation through some form of cognitive appraisal of the immediate situation. Although Schachter and Singer did not describe their model as an attributional conception, subsequent theorists have viewed it in large part as such a conception (see London & Nisbett, 1974).

In a classic investigation designed to test this model, Schachter and Singer (1962) gave some subjects epinephrine, an activating agent, and no information about the arousing effects of the agent. Another group of subjects was given epinephrine and valid information about its effects, while others were given misinformation or not informed about its effect. A final group (nonaroused) was given a saline injection and was not told what to expect from the injection. After the injection, subjects were exposed to an experimental accomplice who was acting in an angry or euphoric manner. The extent to which subjects imitated the accomplice was recorded, as were subjects' ratings of their emotions. Table 2.1 presents means for emotional behavior for the conditions just described.

TABLE 2.1. Effects of physiological arousal and information about arousal on emotional behavior (adapted from Schachter & Singer, 1962).

State of arousal	Accomplice's behavior	
	Euphoric	Angry
Nonaroused (saline-injected)	16.0	0.8
Physiologically aroused (epinephrine-injected)		
Informed	12.7	−0.2
Ignorant	18.3	2.3
Misinformed	22.6	—

Note. The higher the score, the more euphoria or anger the subjects displayed. An epinephrine-injected, misinformed condition was not run with the angry accomplice.

As expected, subjects in the epinephrine-ignorant and epinephrine-misinformed groups imitated the accomplice more than did subjects in the epinephrine-informed condition; also, these subjects rated their emotions as consistent with the accomplice's apparent emotional states. Presumably, subjects in the former conditions were aroused, had no appropriate explanation for their arousal, observed the accomplice's emotional behavior, and concluded that this emotion applied to them too. Subsequent work (e.g., Valins, 1966) has shown that individuals' mere belief that they are aroused is sufficient along with contextual information (e.g., observing the accomplice's emotional behavior) to lead to an attribution of emotion.

Maslach's and Marshall and Zimbardo's Critiques

The work of Schachter and Singer (1962) has been called into question by Maslach (1979) and Marshall and Zimbardo (1979). Maslach suggested that Schachter and Singer's position is weak because people's search for a cognitive explanation of an arousal state is more extensive than Schachter and Singer assumed and biased toward negative emotional labels. She further argued that the drug injection procedure used by Schachter and Singer was flawed because of imprecise control of timing and magnitude of arousal. In a modified replication of their procedure, using hypnosis instead of drug injection, Maslach manipulated whether or not subjects experienced unexplained arousal in the presence of an experimental accomplice who was displaying either happy or angry emotions. Maslach also carried out an exact replication of Schachter and Singer's procedure. She found that subjects with unexplained arousal reported negative emotions regardless of the accomplice's mood. Maslach concluded that a lack of explanation about arousal biases a person's search toward negative emotion. She emphasized that this conclusion differs from Schachter and Singer's view that the lack of explanation leads to an unbiased search. A final finding of note was that subjects' behavior was sociable when the accomplice acted happy. Since subjects' reported emotions were negative, Maslach argued that this sociable behavior was "managed" so as to be socially acceptable in that setting.

Marshall and Zimbardo (1979) replicated and extended Schachter and Singer's procedure. Like Maslach, they too found that unexplained arousal produced negatively toned reports of affect. Further, negative affect was produced merely by the expectation of epinephrine side effects. Unlike Schachter and Singer, Marshall and Zimbardo found no evidence that subjects with inadequately explained epinephrine-produced arousal were more susceptible than placebo controls to the induction of affect by exposure to an accomplice who modeled euphoric behavior. Contrary to Schachter and Singer, Marshall and Zimbardo concluded that there is a lack of "emotional plasticity" in the procedure involving unexplained epinephrine-produced arousal. They also concluded that this type of arousal is associated with negative affect. Overall, Maslach and Marshall and Zimbardo argued that awareness of one's strong arousal without adequate explanation is most likely to be interpreted as a negative mood state.

This discussion would not be complete without brief consideration of Schachter and Singer's (1979) commentary on these critiques. They concluded that pronounced differences in Maslach's procedure (especially regarding timing of emotional experience and when information is given regarding the emotion to be expected) render her work and data noncomparable to their own. As for the Marshall and Zimbardo work, Schachter and Singer also argued that there were such substantial differences in the two studies that no clear comparative conclusions can be drawn. Overall, they claimed that their critics have overlooked a large body of literature that reveals considerable emotional "plasticity" associated with unexplained arousal. Interestingly, Schachter and Singer also concluded that given contemporary ethical guidelines for human research, it is unlikely that ever again will anyone do experiments such as theirs and those by Maslach and Marshall and Zimbardo. In essence, they are suggesting that the plasticity issue in this research paradigm may forever remain inconclusive.

Zillmann's Analysis

Zillmann (1978, 1983) pointed out that according to Schachter and Singer's conception, an emotion cannot be experienced until an excitatory state materializes, is recognized, and is labeled. Zillmann contended that this conception failed to explain why the individual responds in an aroused fashion to certain stimulus conditions in the first place. Rather, as Zillmann argued, the Schachter–Singer approach simply presupposes that cognitive or situational factors trigger physiological processes, and it then deals with what happens after the individual becomes aware of these processes. Zillmann, thus, concluded that this approach is incomplete because it does not address the very origin of an emotional reaction. He suggested that Schachter and Singer had developed a theory that applies only to the emotional experience of people who have developed the skills necessary to engage in full-fledged attributional search activities.

Zillmann's (1978, 1983) own approach was designed to eliminate the shortcoming of the Schachter–Singer approach. Zillmann introduced a three-component model that emphasizes: (a) a *dispositional* component responsible for immediate, motoric emotional reaction (e.g., shaking or blushing), without interpretive activity; (b) an *excitatory* component that energizes behavior because of unconditioned or learned habits (this is the heightened arousal state of the organism); and (c) an *experiential* component which involves the conscious experience of either the motor or the excitatory reaction, or both; it involves an appraisal or attributional element.

Zillmann indicated that after the dispositional motoric response, the excitatory reaction can be seen as preparing the individual to act on the situation so as to avert a potential threat. No attributional search by the individual is conceived to be necessary to find an appropriate explanation for this reaction. Search behavior is seen to be forced upon the individual, especially in ambiguous response situations. In such situations, both dispositional and excitatory reactions are posited to be mediated by the attributional element of the experiential component of emotion.

Zillmann has reviewed diverse evidence, including work on aggression (e.g., Zillmann & Cantor, 1976) and sexual excitement (e.g., Cantor, Zillmann, & Bryant, 1975) as supportive of the three-factor model. In general, Zillmann argued that people in emotional situations often do make attributions but that they may do so in a sporadic, noncontinuous way. He implied that people may "overreact" emotionally in very primitive ways with little or no thought involved (e.g., "This guy is crazy," "You S.O.B.," "Boy, I'll get you for this") and that such overreactions are not interpretable in attributional terms.

Overall, Zillmann's analysis is an elaborate analysis of emotional behavior that promises to be a stimulant for broader and more rigorous work on the role of attribution in the production of emotion. The analysis is, however, so complex that empirical work designed to probe its features may be slow in developing, and thus the analysis may not have the type of immediate impact associated with Schachter and Singer's initial work. What work has been done has, for the most part, examined potential conditions under which cognitive appraisal (attributions) is involved in arousal and emotional processes and the accuracy of such appraisals (Hansen, Hansen, & Crano, in press; Reisenzein & Gattinger, 1982).

A Brief Commentary on the Significance of These Qualifications and Extensions

The qualifications and extensions reviewed in this chapter represent the major theoretical movements in the attribution area after the early foundation work reviewed in chapter 1 (with the exception of Schachter and Singer's work which, as noted above, was not originally conceived as an attributional model). They reveal the great breadth and flexibility of attributional analysis applied in varying contexts and to varying types of human action. They reveal in a clear and major way the impact attributional theorizing has had upon social psychology. These qualifications and extensions were borne out of the early theoretical work, but they, too, have now led to extensive research and writing.

On the other hand, these and other recent qualifications and extensions have been criticized because they represent too little of an advance beyond the early theoretical work. For example, Jones and Kelley (1978) emphasized the fact that numerous attributional theories had emerged but that little theoretical work on basic psychological processes involved in attributions had been done. Essentially, they argued there had been too much application of earlier ideas and development of minitheories for various phenomena and too little work on fundamental processes (as is found in Jones & Davis, 1965, and Kelley, 1967). A number of other criticisms also have surfaced, particularly regarding this work during the 1970s. Critics have said that basic terms were not agreed upon in the area (e.g., the internal–external dichotomy used by many and the endogenous–exogenous dichotomy used by a few—see Shaver, 1979), that the area is a melange or patchwork of diffuse ideas and strands of work.

We will not attempt to analyze the merit of these and other criticisms of developments in the attribution area in the 1970s. As was argued at the beginning of the book, the area is vast in number of ideas, investigators, assumptions about science, beliefs about where work is necessary, and so on. Consensus is not likely to emerge readily among so many workers and so many interested readers. We do think that the basic process problem is now (in the late 1980s) being redressed, and that some of the inconsistencies and controversies have been argued to the point that the strengths and weaknesses of the positions are fairly apparent. Hence, we believe that there will be another season of major theoretical advances in the 1980s and 1990s, and such advances may occur in the context of continuing provocative applications of attribution ideas to address a variety of human problems. Some of this work will be reviewed in the next chapter. As Kelley (1978) said when asked about the past and future of attribution work:

. . . it wasn't some bright idea that somebody had, that somebody forced on somebody's data or tried to extend by brute force. It came out of a lot of phenomena that social psychologists have looked at and tried to interpret. I just can't imagine that the phenomena that are hooked into that kind of cognition will change or be modified. They'll never go away. We'll always have to have that kind of explantion" (p. 384).

3
Theoretical Advances

As we noted in chapter 1, Heider's (1958) analysis of social perception and phenomenal causality stressed the interaction of perceptual and cognitive processes in attribution. Indeed, he argued that in some cases causal information may be inherent in the perceptual organization of information as determined by the properties of the perceptual apparatus. In other cases, he contended, causal information may arise from more deliberative, inferential processes within the perceiver.

Despite Heider's emphasis on *perceived* and *inferred* causality, the early theoretical work (e.g., Jones & Davis, 1965; Jones & McGillis, 1976; Kelley, 1967, 1973) of the late 1960s and early 1970s focused exclusively on the cognitive processes underlying attributional phenomena. As we have seen, the early theorists were concerned with the manner in which individuals analyze information patterns and make more or less logical inferences about the causes of their own and others' behaviors. Kelley's (1967) covariation principle and attributional criteria of distinctiveness, consensus, and consistency information (Kelley, 1973), his causal schemata notion (1972a), Jones and Davis's (1965) and Jones and McGillis's (1976) correspondent inference theory all attempt to model the causal inference process.

This early emphasis on deliberative, inferential processes occurring "within the perceiver's head" probably should not be surprising given the cognitive zeitgeist of the time. Indeed, this zeitgeist still is very dominant in the late 1980s, and we will in this chapter review several recent cognitive models of attributional activity. In contrast to the earlier inferential models, the more recent ones rely to a greater degree on an information processing metaphor and, accordingly, are concerned with more molecular cognitive processes (e.g., processes of information encoding, representation, memory, causal reasoning).

In addition to recent models of inferred causality, we also will be able to examine recent work aimed at elucidating basic perceptual processes underlying attributional activities. While such work represents a return to one form of social knowing identified by Heider (perception-based or direct knowing), it had until the last several years not been an active focus of empirical or theoretical inquiry within the attribution domain.

Finally, in this chapter we will address recent works that have called into question assumptions that underlie traditional attribution conceptions. Topics to be discussed include the extent to which people are aware of the factors that influence them in carrying out social behavior, and the extent to which such behavior is not governed by conscious thought processes.

Basic Perceptual Processes[1]

As we noted in the introduction to this chapter, research in the attribution domain has been guided by a cognitive metaphor, and researchers have made considerable progress in identifying the cognitive structures inside the perceiver's head, that is, the rules of inference and information integration that give rise to certain causal inferences (Jones & Davis, 1965; Jones & McGillis, 1976; Kelley, 1972a, 1973). An alternative view of attributional activities focuses not on perceivers' "higher constructive processes," but instead on the nature and identification of the stimulus information that induces various attributions. This latter view has been called the direct perception or ecological perspective (Baron, 1980; Kassin & Baron, 1985; McArthur & Baron, 1983) on social knowing. According to this perspective, there are naturally occurring organizations of stimulus events that directly and spontaneously induce causal attributions. Since no higher order, inferential processes are required for attributions based on such direct perceptual processes, they are assumed to be made quickly and to require relatively little attention and cognitive effort.

In this section we will review two general classes of environmental cues that may lead perceivers to detect directly causal relationships: temporal contiguity and perceptual salience. We also will examine research on the effects of the perceptual organization of information on causal attributions.

Temporal Contiguity

Recall that in chapter 1 we defined cause as an antecedent, or set of antecedents, that is sufficient for the occurrence of an event. This definition makes explicit a very basic principle guiding attributional processes, name-

---

[1] In this chapter, we will be consider both perceptual and cognitive processes underlying attributional analyses. It is important to note, however, that distinctions between perception and cognition are not always clear. Indeed, labeling mental activity as "perception" or "cognition" often is more a matter of theoretical preference since both may involve mental structures that serve to organize or process stimulus information. Here we will use the terms "perception" and "cognition" to distinguish between attribution processes that require going beyond the immediately given stimulus information to a lesser or greater degree, respectively.

ly, that causes precede effects spatially and/or temporally. So basic is this principle that some (Kassin & Baron, 1985; McArthur & Baron, 1983) have argued that perceivers are either biologically or through perceptual learning attuned to information about the contiguity of stimuli. Moreover, it is argued that this information is sufficient to produce a perception of causality, whether or not there is in reality an objective basis for such a perception.

Consider an example. We feel a gust of wind through an open window and immediately hear a door slam shut. Our immediate perception is that the wind caused the door to close. Of course, other causes of this event are equally plausible. The spring on the door hinge may simply have given way, thereby causing the door to slam shut. Still, our direct and phenomenal percept is that the wind caused the door to shut. So compelling is this apparent cause–effect linkage that we in all likelihood will look no further for other plausible causes.

In a series of early studies, Michotte (1963) demonstrated that spatiotemporal contiguity information is sufficient for the perception of physical causality. In his studies, he observed that certain configurations of visual stimuli, usually the movement of two objects, produced the impression of one object "launching," or pushing the other. Subjects in Michotte's studies, for example, observed two square objects. One of the objects (A) moved at a uniform rate from the left-hand side of the screen toward the second object (B) which was stationary. When A made contact with B, A stopped and B moved away in the same direction and approximately the same speed as A had been moving.

Michotte (1963) argued, "The result of this experiment is perfectly clear: The observers see object A push object B and *drive it, throw it forward, cast it, give it impulsion.* The perception is clear; it is A *that makes B proceed, that produces* its movement" (p. 384). Particularly important was the additional finding that the introduction of even a brief interval (one fifth of a second) between the two events (i.e., between the time A contacts B and B then begins to move) eradicated the perception of causality.

We have in Michotte's early studies, then, a simple demonstration of the importance of contiguity cues on perceptions of physical causality. We do not, however, have from Michotte's work any clear evidence that the spatiotemporal-contiguity effects were based on the direct perception of the dynamic configurations of stimuli. They could have been based on acquired knowledge of specific types of cause–effect sequences (i.e., they could have been cognitively mediated).

Such evidence is provided by studies that have examined young children's attribution processes. There are compelling data, for example, that children as young as 3 or 4 years of age (Mendelson & Shultz, 1976) and even infants of 4 to 8 months of age (Leslie, 1982) causally link contiguous events. Since these young children most certainly do not have the cognitive capacities to engage in sophisticated inferential processes and do not have much in the way of learned cause and effect linkages, it is reasonable to argue that the perception of causality is direct and automatic. (For a more extensive discussion of this literature, see Kassin & Baron, 1985.)

Perceptual Salience

While studies investigating the causal implications of contiguity cues have, for the most part, employed films depicting the movements of geometric figures, research on perceptual salience has relied on films of individuals interacting. What in an interaction setting might make a person perceptually salient?

Let's suppose that you arrive for a social gathering at a friend's home. You understood that the party was to be rather informal. Instead, as you enter, you see that your friends are all decked out and that the party is a sit-down-dinner affair. You, in your jeans, will probably feel a bit conspicuous. Indeed, you will be the center of attention.

This example illustrates one cause of perceptual salience. Specifically, a person can be salient relative to the immediate context by being novel (e.g., solo person of that age, sex, race, hair color, clothing, etc.) or by being somehow more figural (e.g., under a spotlight, exhibiting more movement). Additionally, a person can be salient relative to the perceiver's prior knowledge or expectations (by behaving negatively or extremely) or relative to other attentional tasks (e.g., by dominating the visual field) (Fiske & Taylor, 1984).

What are the consequences of being a salient social stimulus? They are several, and they are important. However, here we will focus on only one consequence—the perceptual salience–attribution effect. Research has demonstrated again and again that people who are perceptually salient are seen as more causally potent than others (Fiske & Taylor, 1984; McArthur, 1981). Moreover, their behavior is seen as more diagnostic of their underlying dispositions.

Why does salience have such effects on causal perceptions? A number of cognitive mediators have been proposed. Enhanced memory for salient stimuli, for example, has been proposed as an explanation for the salience–attribution relationship (Fiske, Kenny, & Taylor, 1982). However, a reliable relationship between recall and causal attributions has been hard to document.

An alternative explanation focuses not on higher order cognitive mediators, but on the initial *registration* of perceptual information. McArthur (1980, 1983) has argued that causal attribution to salient stimuli may depend upon visual scanning activity that registers events in units beginning with the more salient stimulus and ending with the less salient stimulus.

In the context of a dynamic social interaction, each person's behavior is typically both cause and effect: Person A reacts to person B and that reaction causes a reaction in B. The power of certain stimuli to draw attention may cause the perceiver to pick up the salient person's influence on the nonsalient person, rather than vice versa. For example, . . . behavior exchanges . . . [may] be perceptually organized into units reflecting the causal influence of the salient actor on the nonsalient actor (O====o) rather than into units reflecting the causal influence of the nonsalient actor on the salient actor (o----O), regardless of who actually begins the interaction (McArthur, 1980, p. 511).

McArthur's thesis that the perceptual organization of a behavioral sequence at the time of registration yields causal attribution to salient persons is intriguing; however, it has yet to be tested directly. Clearly, such research may provide important insights into the perceptual processes underlying causal attributions and may provide, more specifically, an answer to questions regarding the mediator of the perceptual salience–attribution linkage.

Perceptual Unitization

In the preceding section, we noted that there currently are no data regarding the perceptual organization of social interactions involving salient and nonsalient persons. There is, however, a growing body of research concerned more generally with differences in perceptual unitization, or segmentation of a behavior sequence on causal attributions.

Most of this research is based on earlier work conducted by Newtson (1976). Newtson and his colleagues (Newtson, 1973; Newtson, Engquist, & Bois, 1977) suggest that perceivers may actively participate in the organization of observed behavior into meaningful action units and thus actively control the amounts of information extracted from that behavior. Based on an uncertainty reduction model of information processing (Attneave, 1959), Newtson has proposed and found evidence consistent with the notion that by using finer units of perception, individuals literally generate more information and reduce more uncertainty about the meaning of an action sequence by breaking it into smaller units.

The procedure Newtson has used to measure the units of perception is quite straightforward. In his research, Newtson has provided subjects with a button monitored by a computer. As they watch a videotape of an ongoing behavior sequence, they press the button whenever, in their judgment, one meaningful action ends and another one begins. Using this simple procedure, Newtson has demonstrated that differences in the size of the unit that is discriminated produce differences in subjects' confidence about their judgments of the observed behavior. Moreover, he has demonstrated that the technique is highly reliable over a 5-week test–retest interval, both in terms of the number of actions segmented by a subject for a given behavior sequence and in terms of the probability of particular stimulus intervals being used to segment a given sequence into its component actions. Finally, his research has indicated that differences in the perceptual level of analysis of behavior can be produced by experimental instruction (e.g., segment the sequence into the "smallest" ("largest") actions that seem natural and meaningful to you), by motivational variables (e.g., perceiver's needs and observational goals), or by characteristics of the stimulus information (e.g., unexpected information results in the use of finer units).

Recent empirical tests of Newtson's ideas have been directed at examination of the behavior perception–attribution relationship. A number of investigators have found that a higher rate of unitization often results in more dispositional attributions for an observed other's behavior (Deaux & Major, 1977; Newtson, 1973; Wilder, 1978a, 1978b). There probably are a number of reasons for this unitization–dispositional-attribution relationship. At least one of these is the fact that in observation of many behavior sequences, the focal, or figural stimulus commanding the perceiver's attention is the actor's dynamic and to some extent unpredictable behavior; the situational cues often are stable, contextual, and, consequently, not very salient. Therefore, much of the information gained through higher rates of unitization will be relevant to the actor's dispositions.

The possibility that this unitization–attribution relationship might be mediated by differential memory has been examined in a study reported by Lassiter, Stone, and Rogers (in press). These investigators asked subjects to segment the videotaped behavior of a woman into either fine or gross units. Consistent with earlier research, the unitizing instructions were successfully employed by subjects; those who received the fine-unit instructions segmented the behavior sequence into a greater number of meaningful actions than did those who received gross-unit instructions. Also consistent with past findings, Lassiter et al. reported that fine- compared to gross-unit subjects made more dispositional attributions for the woman's behavior. More importantly, fine-unit subjects remembered more action-related details about the woman's behavior than did gross-unit subjects. Thus, Newtson's (1973) assertion that a higher rate of unitization increases the amount of information available to perceivers received direct support. Subsequent analyses indicated, however, that the relationship between rate of unitization and attributions was not mediated by memory. These results, then, offer support for the notion that perceptual organization of a behavior sequence *at the time of registration* may mediate causal attributions.

Basic Cognitive Processes

In contrast, or perhaps more appropriately, complementary to recent attributional research examining the initial registration of stimulus information, there is a growing literature that examines the higher order, cognitive contents and operations that underlie specific attributions (e.g., Ebbesen & Allen, 1979; Hansen, 1985; Hastie, 1981, 1983, 1984; Read, 1984; Schank & Abelson, 1977; E.R. Smith, 1982, 1984; Smith & Miller, 1979;

Taylor & Fiske, 1978; Trope, 1986; Wyer & Carlston, 1979; Zuckerman, Eghrari, & Lambrecht, 1986; Zuckerman & Evans, 1984). It is important to note, before turning to a discussion of this recent work, that there is much diversity and, at the same time, considerable overlap in the cognitive models and investigative methods employed, and the issues addressed. Consequently, arriving at any organization of the many individual strands of work on basic cognitive processes as they influence attributions is a difficult undertaking. However, for ease of presentation we will categorize (oversimplistically, no doubt) this literature in terms of the dominant type of mental structure or structures invoked as explanatory mechanisms. Specifically, in this section we will focus on work guided by script, implicational-schemata, template-matching, and information-processing stage models of attribution processes. We will not be able to provide an account of all the theoretical and empirical work based on such models; instead we will attempt to present prominent exemplars.

Script Models

Scripts are mental structures that contain knowledge about familiar, routinized sequences of actions oriented toward some goal (Schank & Abelson, 1977). Consider the often-cited restaurant script. This script contains knowledge of the typical sequence of goal-related actions such as entering the restaurant, waiting to be seated, ordering, eating, paying, and exiting. It also contains knowledge of typical "actors" and "roles" in this scene— maitre d', waiter, customer, etc. Finally, the restaurant script includes knowledge about "props" that are important for carrying out the action sequence, in this instance, menus, plates, eating utensils, money, etc.

In other words, scripts involve knowledge of "a coherent sequence of events expected by the individual, involving him either as a participant or as an observer" (Abelson, 1976, p. 33). They contain features abstracted from many single vignettes (e.g., the images of an event that has recently occurred), the basic ingredients of scripts that help group similar experiences and also help differentiate contrasting ones. Scripts are important because they influence our perceptions of, memories for, and expectations about (future) events.

Two script models of attribution processes have been proposed by Read (1987) and Hilton and Slugoski (1986). Though differing in important ways, both of these models contend that people use detailed, domain-specific knowledge of normal or usual behavior to construct causal scenarios for social events. They also assert that to understand fully attributional processes, we must understand the content and structure of these scenarios.

More specifically, both models argue that when observed behavior fits an existing script, the script *contains* the explanation for the event. For example, the script contains information relevant to a covariation (a la Kelley) or correspondent inference (a la Jones & Davis) analysis—information about what is high-consensus, socially desirable (information about what is normal) behavior. When observed behavior does not fit the script (low-consensus, socially undesirable behavior), the script provides information about the normal background against which the deviant or abnormal behavior can be explained. Such deviations from scripts instigate a search for causal explanations.

While Read's (1987) general model of attribution processes focuses on the construction and structure of causal scenarios, or scripts for social events, Hilton and Slugoski's (1986) abnormal-conditions model emphasizes attributional complexities arising when events are not instances of scripted behavior or script deviations. According to Hilton and Slugoski, when trying to understand nonscripted social events or sequences, observers treat consensus, distinctiveness, and consistency information as contrast cases that define the abnormal conditions resulting in the production of the target event. The abnormal conditions, then, are identified as the causes of the event. For example, high-consensus information for scripted events ("everyone eats something upon going to this restaurant") is uninformative about the cause of a particular actor's behavior, while such information ("everyone is afraid of this dog") may define an abnormal condition and, hence, cause (an unusually fierce dog) of a nonscripted event.

While Read's (1987) and Hilton and Slugoski's (1986) script models of attribution processes are in some ways related to the early theoretical work of Kelley (1967) and Jones and his colleagues (Jones & Davis, 1965; Jones & McGillis, 1976), there are a number of important differences. Both of these script models focus on extended sequences of behaviors, rather than a single event. Both focus to a greater degree than early formulations on the important role of attributors' extensive social knowledge. Both focus on domain-specific, as opposed to more "content-free" or "procedural" knowledge; examples of the latter type would include Kelley's (1972a) causal-schemata notions that posit the existence of general procedural, or process rules that represent general knowledge about cause–effect linkages that apply across a wide range of content areas (e.g., extreme effects require multiple causes). And, finally, both emphasize the importance of contrastive [as opposed to (Hilton & Slugoski, 1986) or in addition to (Read, 1987)] covariational criteria in causal-inference processes.

Implicational-Schema Models

A script may be viewed as a specific instance of a more general class of mental structures, schemata. A schema may be defined as a cognitive structure that represents an individual's organized knowledge about a given concept or stimulus domain (Fiske & Taylor, 1984). We may, for example, have a "professor" schema. Such a schema would contain our accumulated general knowledge of what constitutes a professor—the relevant attributes and the relationships among these attributes. Or we may have a schema for "honesty" that includes all of the behaviors that are relevant to the concept and the relationships among these behaviors.

The concept of schema is, of course, not new to attribution theory. As we saw in chapter 1, Kelley (1972a) proposed that sometimes attributors use *causal* schemata, which are well-learned patterns of cause and effect relationships, to understand and make meaningful social situations.

Exending this scehemata reasoning, Reeder (Reeder, 1985; Reeder & Brewer, 1979) recently has proposed a schematic model of *dispositional* attribution. This model identifies several general prototype schemata, or classes of implicit assumptions, that may underlie our understanding of various dispositional terms (see Figure 3.1). These assumptions may interact and jointly determine dispositional attributions. The assumptions Reeder identifies as important in the dispositional-attribution process are reinforcement (individuals attempt to vary their behavior to meet situational contingencies), central-tendency (type of behavior most likely to be emitted by individuals with a given disposition), social-desirability (most individuals tend to behave in a socially desirable fashion), and ability (individuals with high ability have a greater range of behavior than those with low ability) assumptions.

More specifically, Reeder's schematic model suggests that observers make certain systematic assumptions about the range of behavior that is implied by a given disposition. These schematic assumptions are thought to influence implicational relations, or implicit links between dispositions and their implied behaviors, which in turn determine the inferred disposition. For example, high intelligence appears to imply that an actor has the capacity to emit both highly intelligent and unintelligent overt behaviors. On the other hand, low intelligence implies that the actor has the ability to perform unintelligently but not intelligently, regardless of situational contingencies and demands. Consequently, when observers witness an overt portrayal of the actor's high ability, dispositional inferences of ability

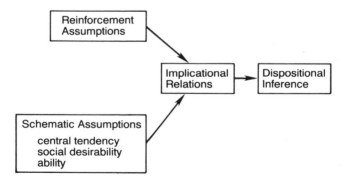

FIGURE 3.1. Schematic model of dispositional attribution.

should be less affected by observation of situational demands than should inferences based on low-ability behavior (Reeder & Fulks, 1980). Reeder and his colleagues (Reeder, Henderson, & Sullivan, 1982; Reeder, Messick, & Van Avermaet, 1977; Reeder & Spores, 1983) have amassed some evidence in support of their general model.

Template-Matching Models

Another class of mental structures includes template schemas. These schemas may be thought of as filing systems for classifying, retaining, and coordinating incoming data (Hastie, 1981). Several authors (Hansen, 1985; Orvis, Cunningham, & Kelley, 1975; Smith & Miller, 1979) have proposed that attributional processing may best be characterized as a template-matching-plus-correction process. Basically, these models suggest that attributors come to a causal quandary with Kelley's (1967) three causal forces (i.e., person, entity, and circumstance) and templates of typical data patterns (high or low consensus, distinctiveness, and consistency) associated with attributions to the three causal forces. Attributors then are thought to attempt a fit of the obtained data with the template. The template that best fits the obtained data pattern determines the causal attribution.

Perhaps the most comprehensive treatment of the template-matching models of attribution has been provided by Hansen (1980, 1985). Hansen bases his model on five propositions:

1. Individuals come to the attribution task with at least three hypothetical causal explanations in mind. Behavior may be seen as facilitated by a force within the actor, a force within the entity, or the circumstances under which the actor is interacting with the entity.
2. Upon observation of a behavioral event, one of these facilitative forces is tentatively advanced as an explanation for the event.
3. This causal guess then guides the perceiver's search for causal information on which to base a more resolute causal explanation for the event.
4. This search for information, as guided by the causal guess, follows a principle of cognitive economy: Rather than search for information allowing for the disconfirmation of alternative explanations, individuals prefer information allowing for simpler confirmatory inferences over information that would permit more complicated confirmatory inferences (inferences based on augmentation or discounting).
5. When the causal guess entails a person attribution, attributors will search for distinctiveness information to validate their guess. When it involves a stimulus or entity attribution, attributors will search for consensus information.

Hansen has provided support for a number of these propositions in a series of five studies. A number of important issues, of course, remain at this point. It is unclear, for example, what determines or constitutes an acceptable level of fit between observed and schematically represented data patterns. It also is unclear whether or how attributors recognize the difference between causal guesses and firmer causal conclusions. This is a particularly important issue since we may often arrive at causal judgments automatically, spontaneously, "off the top of our heads" (Heider, 1958; Taylor & Fiske, 1978).

Evaluation of Schematic Models

An analysis by Fiedler (1982) critically analyzes the attributional-schemata construct and related research. While much of his critique focuses on causal schemata (Kelley, 1972a), many of his points also apply to Reeder's implicational-schemata notion and to script-schema notions. Fiedler argues that to date studies have not been designed to test observable schema properties and that the available research lacks essential features of natural causal problems. Further, Fiedler contends that although an important aspect of natural causal tasks is the encoding of unstructured empirical information, the stimulus materials in a great many schema studies have been prestructured to such a degree that the task left to judge is simply reporting semantic relations. Although Fiedler's analysis should prove helpful in refining the attributional schema construct, it is unclear what effect it will have on empirical research. As we have noted elsewhere (Harvey & Weary, 1984), his request for greater rigor in analysis and, at the same time, greater naturalism in stimulus material could be applied to any area of contemporary social–cognition work.

Information-Processing Models

Probably no discussion of models of higher order constructive processes underlying attributions would be complete without consideration of the currently popular information-processing approaches. Like the schematic models discusssed above, these approaches to causal-inference processes invoke various knowledge structures as important explanatory mechanisms. However, the information-processing models generally consider the cognitive operations hypothesized to occur at each of several processing stages.

A prominent exemplar of the information-processing models of causal inference is that introduced by Hastie (Hastie, 1981; Hastie & Kumar, 1979) and elaborated further by Srull (1981). A flowchart of the hypothesized processing stages in this model is depicted in Figure 3.2.

Briefly, this information-processing model postulates that:

1. During the acquisition stage, propositional representations of each stimulus person's behaviors are formed in memory.
2. When unexpected behaviors are observed, the perceiver is likely to engage in causal reasoning in order to understand why these behaviors

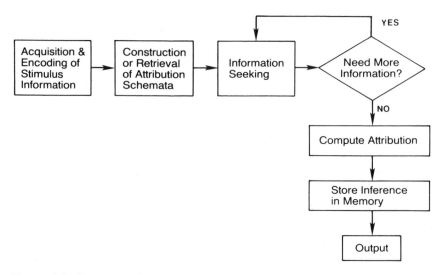

FIGURE 3.2. Sequence of processing stages in causal reasoning. (Adapted from Hastie, 1984.)

    occurred. The construction or retrieval of attributional schemata may characterize processing at this stage.
3. The consequence of this extra causal reasoning is a more elaborate memory representation for the unexpected information and an increased number of associative links between the incongruent behavior and the other behaviors of that stimulus person.
4. The unexpected event, by virtue of this longer or more elaborate processing, will be likelier to be recalled than behaviors that were not unexpected.
5. This greater recall for unexpected events will play a bigger role in the perceiver's subsequent judgments about and behavior toward the stimulus person.

    Evidence consistent with this general model has been found in a series of studies reported by Hastie (1984). However, an examination of diverse literature concerned with the memory-for-events–social-judgment relationship reveals that there are a number of models relevant to this relationship and that it may be far more complex than originally thought. For a more complete treatment of various processing models that relate memory for events and various social judgments, including attributions, readers should see Hastie and Park (1986).

Concluding Points

While relatively recent introductions to the attribution domain, the schematic and information-processing models (Hastie, 1981; Smith, 1984;

Trope, 1986) hold the promise of contributing to our understanding of basic cognitive processes involved in self- and other-attributions and the role of causal inference processes in person memory, more generally.

However, they are not without problems. Often the cognitive-stage formulations are little more than loose frameworks for an information-processing theory, not specific, working models (for a notable exception see Trope's, 1986, mathematical model that decomposes the attribution of personal dispositions into stages of identification and dispositional-inferential processes); consequently, multiple models tend to fit the available data. Indeed, it often appears that knowledge structures like scripts and schemas are post hoc interpretations of data that are one step removed from data description (Zuckerman, Eghrari, & Lambrecht, 1986). Additionally, many of the models and supporting data have been imported from other domains, primarily from work on language comprehension. While the analogy from semantic to social memory may be an appropriate one, it does seem that much more empirical work using more naturalistic stimulus materials (rather than or in addition to linguistic materials) to represent social stimuli and events will be necessary to demonstrate this. Finally, few of the models of cognitive processes of attribution deal in any substantial way with the very early stages of information acquisition. Exactly how and what stimulus information gets registered and then cognitively operated upon is a question that badly needs some attention. It seems possible that some integration of the work discussed in this chapter on basic perceptual processes with the social cognition approaches might take us a long way in terms of developing more comprehensive, process models of attribution.

One final comment is probably worth making here. A return to basic attributional-process issues such as we have seen during the 1980s surely is long overdue. However, we often have heard that the social-cognition models that are so popular today and indeed are so important have supplanted Heider's less precise depiction of the cognitions underlying interpersonal relations. We would like to argue, however, that the attribution approaches, on the one hand, and the social-cognition approaches, on the other, are dealing with different levels of analysis, and we are sure that there is room and need for both. Indeed, an adequate understanding of interpersonal relations would seem to require both. Like Olson and Ross (1985), we

... value the unique qualities of the attribution approach. Social cognition researchers have, for the most part, restricted their attention to cognitive phenomena, staying "within the head" of the perceiver. In contrast, attribution researchers have increasingly incorporated affective and behavioral measures into their studies and have moved their research into dynamic, interpersonal settings. As a consequence, we believe that the attribution literature holds promise for becoming a true "*social* psychology of interpersonal cognition", both distinct from and complementary to social cognition's cognitive emphasis (p. 305).

Critical Analyses of Attribution Assumptions

In the remainder of this chapter, we will address the question of how aware people are of the various and often complex attributions they make about others—especially significant others—in their lives. How aware is Bob that after 6 weeks of dating Sally he has developed an interpretation of Sally as an arrogant, selfish person who is never likely to be very good for him? Are people sometimes highly deliberate and thoughtful in making these attributions (as, for example, Kelley, 1967, would suggest)? Or are they only somewhat deliberate and *aware* (as Kelley, 1972a, would suggest)? Or are they very much unaware, as some of the theorists to be mentioned in this chapter might suggest? A conclusion that we will foster in this section is that each of these possibilities may be true under certain conditions. The important task is to discover those conditions.

We should make it clear from the outset that the most imposing analyses to be discussed below apply to theories in cognitive social psychology, generally. As they picture humans to be thoughtful and deliberate, most theories in this general domain would be subject to challenge by the principal analyses to be discussed. However, attributional theories and constituent assumptions are at the center of contemporary cognitive social psychology and, hence, represent a major target of these critical analyses.

Awareness of Cognitive Processes and Influencing Variables

An analysis about people's cognitive shortcomings was presented by Nisbett and Wilson (1977). These theorists were concerned about how thoughtful people indeed are in making attributions and predictions, forming judgments, and so on. In fact, they were quite skeptical about traditional conceptions regarding people's rather ample capabilities. Nisbett and Wilson offered three general arguments that may be paraphrased from their statement (p. 233) as follows:

1. People often cannot report accurately on the effects of particular stimuli on higher order, inference based responses. Further, they sometimes cannot report on critical stimuli that affect them, their responses to such stimuli, or the processes (such as attribution) intervening between stimuli and responses. Nisbett and Wilson say, "The accuracy of subjective reports is so poor as to suggest that any introspective access that may exist is not sufficient to produce generally correct or reliable reports" (p. 233).
2. When reporting on the effects of stimuli, people may not use a memory of the intervening cognitive processes that were influenced by the stimuli. Rather, they may base their reports on implicit, causal theories about the connection between stimulus and response. These theories are simi-

lar to causal schemata in Kelley's (1972a) analysis. For example, "They had that terrible fight because she had had a rough day, and he then came home and pestered her." This attribution corresponds generally to a multiple-cause schema people might hold for explaining "terrible fights." According to Nisbett and Wilson, there are various other types of implicit causal theories, and they mostly are ideas we learn to hold through our daily experiences and societal norms.

3. Finally, subjective reports about higher mental processes are sometimes correct, but even the instances of accuracy are not due to introspective awareness. Instead, these correct reports are due to the incidentally correct employment of a priori causal theories such as those mentioned above.

Before discussing Nisbett and Wilson's position further, and criticisms of that position, a number of general comments about the analysis are necessary. First, it is notable that Nisbett and Wilson seem to be adopting an "anti-introspectionist" position (Rich, 1979). Arguments favoring either introspection or anti-introspection positions frequently were presented in the early part of the 20th century when the science of psychology was being developed. While such arguments have not been so common in recent years, Nisbett and Wilson have helped rekindle interest in the role of introspection in experimental psychology. Not unlike Bem's (1967b, 1972) well-known arguments, Nisbett and Wilson's analysis is a stirring polemical work that involves *a degree* of logical and empirical support and that has received notice throughout the field of psychology.

The general import of Nisbett and Wilson's analysis for attribution conceptions derives from the fact that many of the major conceptions (e.g., Heider, 1958; Jones & Davis, 1965; Kelley, 1967) at least imply awareness, and probably some degree of accuracy, in people's attributional activities in terms of their knowledge of what general factors are affecting them and how they are responding on a behavioral and cognitive level. It is important to note, however, that the major attributional formulations do not imply that there is complete awareness or a high degree of accuracy. Very definitely, Nisbett and Wilson are arguing for a limited attributional capacity on the part of the human organism. Also, they are arguing that what attributional activity does occur is not as thoughtful and extemporaneous as has been suggested in most major theoretical statements.

Before reviewing criticisms of Nisbett and Wilson's position, let us examine briefly a study that is illustrative of the evidence they cite (see also Wilson, 1985) as supportive of their arguments regarding the limited accessibility of mental states. In a study by Nisbett and Schachter (1966), subjects were requested to take a series of electric shocks of steadily increasing intensity. Before being exposed to the shock, some of the subjects were given a placebo pill which, they were told, would produce various arousal symptoms such as heart palpitations. Nisbett and Schachter expected that when subjects with these instructions were exposed to the shock, they would attribute their arousal symptoms to the pill and thus would tolerate more shock than would subjects who could only attribute these symptoms to the shock. This expectation was strongly borne out in the results. After subjects participated, they were interviewed to see if they could explain their tendencies to take more or lesser degrees of shock. They reported little awareness. This unawareness held even when placebo pill subjects were asked if they thought the pill was causing some effects. Only 3 out of 12 subjects reported having made the postulated attributions of arousal to the pill, and in general the subjects did not believe they had followed the thought sequence specified by the hypothesis when it was explained to them.

Nisbett and Wilson used this evidence, as well as results from other studies to suggest that generally no association has been found between the degree of verbal report change and degree of behavior change in experimental groups. Their argument is intriguing. However, a number of questions about the argument have been raised (Bowers, 1979; Rich, 1979; Smith & Miller, 1978; White, 1980).

Smith and Miller (1978) suggested that Nisbett and Wilson's position cannot be readily refuted or properly tested. According to Smith and Miller, Nisbett and Wilson appear to regard as illustrative of their position both correct and incorrect accounts by subjects of their reasoning processes. As Smith and Miller noted, the Nisbett–Wilson argument consists in part of a series of studies in which subjects are unable to report the influence of effective stimulus factors. But as Smith and Miller contended, "Nisbett and Wilson . . . are implicitly using an impossible criterion for introspective awareness: that subjects be aware of what we systematically and effectively hide from them by our experimental design . . . a between-subjects design . . . makes it impossible for the subject to know what is being experimentally varied and what is being held constant" (p. 256). White (1980) essentially reinforced these methodological criticisms and provided further arguments about the insensitivity of the methods Nisbett and Wilson employed.

Bowers's (1979) commentary is perhaps the most potent of the critical analyses of Nisebett and Wilson's thesis. In addition to touching on points such as those mentioned above, Bowers argues that if the causes of behavior are necessarily and automatically as accessible to people as they in fact are influential in affecting behavior, then there would be no need for psychology. People would, in such a case, know all that there is to know about human behavior; hence, why would we need to investigate human behavior? The answer to this rhetorical but compelling line of reasoning is that people cannot possibly always know the causes of their behavior. They may have an understanding that more or less parallels that of the scientist. But even the scientist's causal understanding is probably incomplete and subject to revision. Thus, in this conception, Nisbett and Wilson's curiosity about people's limitations regarding introspective access to understanding of their behavior is puzzling—how could people not be so limited? Bower's analysis also leads to a stance that Nisbett and Wilson may have developed some leads about a theory of the unconscious determinants of behavior. Bowers recommends a continuation of that development that will likely involve examination of a question stated early in this discussion, namely: When and why are people highly aware, less aware, or not aware of the influences on their behavior?

Recently, Wilson (1985) has turned his attention to just such questions. He argues that individuals may lack access not only to the causes of behavior, but also to mental states (attitudes, moods, traits, evaluations) more generally. He proposes a cognitive process model that involves two mental systems: one that mediates behavior and is largely nonconscious, and one that is conscious and functions to verbalize and explain behavior. Wilson identifies several conditions under which individuals may have access to their mental states; under such conditions, the verbal system can make direct and accurate reports. When there is limited access, however, Wilson argues that the verbal system makes "guesses," or inferences about what these states may be. Such guesses may be incorrect and may conflict with unregulated behavioral indices of the psychological state.

Concluding Points

As we have seen in this section, challenges to basic attribution assumptions have evolved from arguments concerning people's cognitive limitations. These challenges relate to notions that individuals often lack awareness of their thought processes and are inaccurate in reporting their mental states.

Wilson's (1985) proposal of two cognitive systems is interesting and has received some modest support. Specifically, in a series of studies, Wilson and his colleagues (Wilson, Hull, & Johnson, 1981; Wilson & Linville, 1982) have found evidence consistent with the notion that priming can affect the verbal but not the behavioral system. There are a number of thorny, theoretical issues, however, that will be difficult to address empirically. It will, for example, be quite difficult to test issues of accuracy of one or both systems since criteria of accuracy are most difficult to come by. Clearly additional theoretical and empirical work is necessary before further advances will occur in our understanding of people's awareness of their own mental processes.

4
Developmental Aspects of the Attributional Process

In the preceding chapters, discussions focused on the attributions of adults. Although such emphasis is natural, given the subject populations traditionally studied, it must not blind us to the possibility that adult attributions are part of a developmental progression and therefore differ from the attributional activity of young children. This chapter explores various attempts to address that issue and to specify developmental patterns in the process of attributing responsibility and causality. The chapter is based on Harris (1981) which was included in the earlier edition of this text. However, we have modified and extended Harris's (1981) work to include more recent empirical studies and theoretical conceptions.

The conceptual distinction between causality and responsibility was reviewed in chapter 1. Shaver (1985), in a recent book on the assignment of blame, discussed this distinction at great length and proposed a further conceptual differentiation between the assignment of responsibility and blame. While both terms refer to attributions for negative outcomes, the latter involves attributional disagreement between the actor and perceiver. Shaver (1985) suggested that blame usually occurs when an actor has provided some excuse or justification for a negative outcome that a perceiver disbelieves. Shaver elaborated upon these distinctions and proposed a theory of blame incorporating a sequence of judgments that occur after a negative event. Namely, attributions of causality precede judgments of responsibility which in turn elicit excuses and justifications from the actor for his/her behavior. The latter are then evaluated by a perceiver and blame is assigned to the actor accordingly.

As Shaver (1985) noted, distinctions between the assignment of blame and responsibility have not been made consistently in the developmental literature. Responsibility and causality generally have been considered separately, however, and therefore will be covered independently within the current chapter. In this chapter, we will include discussion of developmental aspects of Heider's (1958) theory, attributionally relevant aspects of Piaget's moral development theory, and empirical research generated by these theoretical statements. We also will review recent developmental studies of Kelley's (1967, 1972b) covariation and discounting principles, as well as research addressing the related overjustification effect (Lepper, Greene, & Nisbett, 1973). Another body of developmental literature investigating achievement-related attributions will be reviewed in chapter 9.

Noteworthy research also has been conducted on the development of trait attributions (e.g., Calveric, 1979; Guttentag & Longfellow, 1978; Livesley & Bromley, 1974) and the relationship between parents' attributions and children's behavior (e.g., Bugental, 1987; Dix & Grusec, 1985). However, these topics will not be reviewed in this chapter.

The Attribution of Responsibility and Blame

As noted above, distinctions between responsibility and blame have not been a focus of developmental research (Shaver, 1985). In fact, none of the developmental work to be reviewed here specifically addresses the concept of blame as defined by Shaver (1985). Rather, studies for the most part have considered the terms responsibility and blame as interchangeable, with both assessed by any questions regarding an actor's naughtiness, blame, or responsibility for some event. Hence, the work to be reviewed here has in common two elements: (a) use of developmental populations and (b) evaluations of blame, naughtiness, or responsibility of an actor involved in some event.

The majority of work in this area developed out of two major theoretical perspectives—Piaget's theory of moral development and Heider's developmental conception of responsibility attribution. Research that has developed from these perspectives will be considered separately, but the reader should keep in mind that both bodies of literature have attempted to elucidate developmental patterns of responsibility attributions and moral judgments.

The Moral Judgment Paradigm of Jean Piaget

Piaget's work, *The Moral Judgment of the Child* (1932), has had a major influence on the study of developmental patterns of responsibility attribution. Methodologically, Piaget's technique of eliciting children's attributions to story characters continues to be a feature of recent moral judgment studies. Theoretically, Piaget's writing on moral development has been equally influential. In it, he describes children's progression from a stage of generally *egocentric morality* to the more relative *morality of reciprocity* (Hoffman, 1970). In these two stages, the moral judgments of children are predicted to differ in many ways. However, the most relevant aspect of Piaget's theory for attribution theory concerns children's transition from objective to subjective evaluations of social behavior. According to Piaget, a young child's judgment of the correctness or incorrectness of an act is based on the external, or objective characteristics of the actor's behavior (e.g., how much damage is caused by an act). Conversely, in the more mature stage of subjective responsibility children's judgments are based on internal attributes such as intentionality (e.g., how much did the actor intend for a certain outcome to occur).

To test children's use of objective versus subjective attributes in moral judgments, Piaget designed a number of story pairs. One story within each pair contained an act based on good intent that caused significant damage, while the second story involved an act based on negative intent (disobedience) that caused a small amount of damage. To illustrate, we present one of Piaget's story pairs (1932, p. 86):

Good intent/high damage [Story IA]: A little boy who is called John is in his room. He is called to dinner. He goes into the dining room. But behind the door there was a chair, and on the chair there was a tray with fifteen cups on it. John couldn't have known that there was all this behind the door. He goes in, the door knocks against the tray, bang go the fifteen cups and they all get broken.

Bad intent/low damage [Story IB]: Once there was a little boy whose name was Henry. One day when his mother was out he tried to get some jam out of the cupboard. He climbed up on to a chair and stretched out his arm. But the jam was too high up and he couldn't reach it and have any. But while he was trying to get it he knocked over a cup. The cup fell down and broke.

After hearing each pair of stories, children were asked to state which child was the naughtier of the two. Piaget reasoned that if responsibility (or blame) were judged by objective criteria (indicating a less mature stage), the child in the high-damage story should be judged naughtier. The children tested ranged from 6 to 10 years of age, and Piaget found that as age increased, there was a gradual shift from objective to subjective judgments.

Evaluation of Piaget's Paradigm

From an attributional perspective, Piaget's work (1932) was both provocative and frustratingly incomplete. It was provocative in its suggestion that adults' interest in dispositional attributes (Heider, 1944; Ross, 1977) might not be shared by attributors of all ages. The frustration, however, came from Piaget's failure to specify the precise mechanism(s) responsible for this effect. This failure stemmed largely from the fact that the story pairs confounded outcome and intention—that is, low damage was always associated with negative intent and high damage with good intent. Thus, if a child judged John to be naughtier than Henry (Story IA vs. IB above), it was impossible to say whether this was due to John's (good) intention being ignored or to the extensive negative outcome of his door opening (the breaking of 15 cups). From this work, one could assume any one of at least three different interpretations: (a) children could not differentiate intentionality from unintentionality; (b) they were able to differentiate the two, but did not use intentionality to judge naughtiness; (c) they differentiated and used intentionality as would adults, but intentionality was not clearly contained in Piaget's stories (e.g., reaching for jam was not a clearly malintentioned act).

Recent Studies of Moral Evaluation

Fortunately, the methodological problems with Piaget's work have been acknowledged widely (see Imamoglu, 1976; Karniol, 1978; Keasey, 1978), and there have been many attempts to modify the basic Piagetian paradigm (see Keasey, 1978, for a review of studies within this paradigm). The primary goal of these modifications has been to assess more directly children's attention to intentionality in social events using a variety of populations, stimulus measures, and dependent measures. The focus also has moved away from the more descriptive approach used by Piaget (e.g., asking, what conclusions do children make?) toward more systematic examination of how children use information to reach specific conclusions (e.g., what decision rules do children use?) (Shultz & Kestenbaum, 1985).

The basic plan of these more recent studies was evident in Armsby's "reexamination of the developments of moral judgments in children" (1971). The most important feature of this study was the author's independent manipulation of intention and outcome. Separate stories containing either unintentional or intentional acts were constructed. Each act also was paired with one of four different amounts of damage (e.g., breaking one cup, 15 cups, all the plates in the house, or a television). A second noteworthy feature of Armsby's method was his care in making the damage-causing act itself the locus of the actor's intentionality or unintentionality—something not done by Piaget or by many contemporary researchers (see Karniol, 1978, on this point).

Using these simple modifications of Piaget's paradigm, Armsby found the same developmental trend as did Piaget (increasing use of intention) but at a much earlier age: a full 75% of the sample of 6-year-olds based their attributions of naughtiness on the subjective attribute of intentionality. Subsequent research on the attribution of intention has generally supported Armsby's findings, while also exploring the effects of certain stimulus variables and methodological refinements. One such variable is the mode by which stimulus events are presented. In most of the literature, experimenters presented stories orally or in written form (e.g., Armsby, 1971). Stimulus events also have been acted out and presented either on film (King, 1971) or on videotape (e.g., Farnill, 1974), with videotaped stories sometimes producing more intention-based attributions than stories which were read to subjects (Chandler, Greenspoon, & Barenboim, 1973; Shultz & Butkowsky, 1977). These data imply that more "realistic" stories elicited greater adult-like attributions in children. Other studies, however, have failed to replicate this finding (Brendt & Brendt, 1975).

A second variation in methodology concerns the way in which subjects' attributions were elicited. Although many experiments followed the Piagetian tradition of forced-choice selection from multiple pairs of stimulus stories, some asked subjects to rate the goodness or badness of actors in individual stories (e.g., Costanzo, Coie, Grumet, & Farnill, 1973). While there is reason to believe that such a procedure might change subjects' patterns of attribution, the evidence on this point is ambiguous (Berg-Cross, 1975; see Keasey, 1978, for a discussion).

A third methodological issue involves memory of intention information versus information about outcome. If youngest children have the most trouble coding story events (Copple & Coon, 1977), it is reasonable to think that their memory might show a recency effect. Thus, they might selectively remember more outcome-relevant information since it is usually presented last (see Piaget's stories above). Evidence supporting this idea was found by Nummedal and Bass (1976), and many experimenters attempted to minimize such memory-based artifacts by giving children pictorial or written summaries of stimulus events (e.g., Armsby, 1971). Children also at times have been asked to repeat the story until it was retold accurately (e.g., Fincham, 1981).

Effects of Outcome Valence and Severity

With methodological refinements discussed above, it has become possible to validate and test independently for the effects of intention and outcome on moral judgments. As already noted, the use of information about others' intentions was exhibited by children as young as 6 years old (given the right conditions), and seemed to increase slightly with age. There has been a fairly recent controversy, however, regarding the impact of outcome valence on this pattern of results. Although assignment of responsibility or blame presupposes a negative outcome valence, we will review the effects of outcome valence in general in order to examine responsibility attributions within the larger context of moral evaluation.

Early research indicated that children incorporated intention information into moral evaluations or attributions at an earlier age when the outcome was positive rather than negative (Costanzo et al., 1973; Farnill, 1974). Costanzo et al. (1973), for example, reported that children as young as 5 years old rated actors in scenarios with positive consequences more positively when they were described as having good intentions rather than bad intentions. On the other hand, 5-year-olds who heard stories with negative outcomes failed to incorporate intentions into moral judgments. However, as age increased, so did children's use of intention information under negative outcome conditions. Costanzo and Dix (1983), in a review of this work, suggested that these differential patterns may have resulted from different socialization patterns implemented by parents in response to acts with positive and negative outcomes.

Parents may become upset by any act that creates a negative outcome, regardless of their child's intentions, but may reward acts with positive outcomes only when they are well-intentioned. Under these differential reinforcement conditions, a child may learn the importance of intention in receiving praise for positive outcomes before realizing the impact of intention on getting blamed for a negative outcome. For example, a child who is scolded every time he drops and breaks a dish, regardless of whether he did so on purpose, will have difficulty learning that "doing it on purpose" sometimes gets one in more trouble. Likewise, if a child is praised for carrying his dishes safely from the table to the sink only when it is clear from a parent's reminder or a child's statement that intention not to break the dish was operating, he/she will learn quickly the value of *trying* to carry out acts that will produce positive outcomes.

The suggestion that intention information is used at an earlier age when outcomes are positive was challenged by Fincham (1983a, 1985a). He reported that young children in his studies made judgments of an actor's "kindness or naughtiness" in line with those made by adults only when outcome valence was negative. Specifically, both 5-year-old children and adults judged actors who behaved spontaneously to be naughtier than actors who performed a behavior under conditions of obedience or reciprocity, although the degree to which this pattern occurred increased with age. (These results corroborated earlier data from Armsby, 1971.) On the other hand, when outcome valence was positive, only adults judged spontaneous actors to be kinder than constrained actors. Shultz, Wright, and Schleifer (1986) also reported that 5-year-olds used intention information when assigning punishment (probably a reflection of blame) for behaviors that had resulted in negative outcomes.

These conflicting stances regarding the influence of outcome valence are difficult to sort out. Although variations in experimental procedures across laboratories may account for some of the differences, the full impact of outcome valence probably cannot be assessed thoroughly without consideration of the severity/intensity of the outcome in question. It may be, for example, that young children only use intention in their moral evaluations of acts which lead to excess or severe damage. In fact, some studies demonstrated that the effect of outcome severity on moral judgments decreased with age (e.g., Armsby, 1971; Keasey, 1978). In a more recent paper by Fincham (1982a), outcome severity influenced moral attributions made even by adults. Hence, the existing data do not provide clear evidence regarding the relationship between outcome valence, severity, and attributions of moral responsibility.

Concluding Points

Piaget's theory of moral development has been the impetus for a significant amount of work regarding children's evaluations of responsibility and blame (although again, these terms have not been differentiated appropriately according to Shaver). In general the work has supported Piaget's theory, demonstrating developmental increases in the use of intention when judging the naughtiness of an actor's behavior. Refinements in the theory have been suggested, however, most often based on attribution patterns that vary with methodological differences in the mode of stimulus presentation, methods of assessing attribution, and valence and severity of outcomes.

To our knowledge, the literature has not been extensive in addressing the impact that these attributional patterns have on subsequent social interactions or affective responses in children or adults. As will be evident in chapter 9, relationships between attribution and affect have been examined within an achievement context, and some work has attempted to expand these linkages beyond that context (e.g., Graham & Weiner, 1986). However, within the domain of moral evaluation, it would be of interest to know how children's responsibility attributions of peers' behaviors influence their own behavior toward peers, the affective responses and behavior of the peers, and adult observers' reactions. Examination of questions such as these could help place the process of blame assignment within the broader context of developmental social interactions. Such a paradigm has been applied, for example, in an attempt to examine the role of children's attributions in psychotherapy treatment outcome (Braswell, Koehler, & Kendall, 1985).

Heider's Concept of Attributed Responsibility

Research on Piaget's subjective/objective distinction identified intentionality of an action as its most developmentally significant attribute. Although intentionality is an important cue for making social attributions, there is no reason to assume that other characteristics of an event are not equally important. For example, Heider's (1958) theory of interpersonal attribution (see chap. 1) involves identification of both personal and environmental attributes that affect judgments of causality and responsibility. In this more general vein, Heider also speculated on possible developmental trends in the utilization of these causal attributes.

The developmental aspect of Heider's theory suggested that observers' judgments of an actor's responsibility for an event should show an age-related developmental progression. Five specific levels of responsibility, each based on different combinations of personal and environmental forces, were described by Heider (1958) as follows:

I. The first level was that of *association*, marked by the attribution of responsibility to a person "P" for any event with which he was in any way associated. For example, a person named Fred could be held responsible for an event caused in his presence or for an act unknown to him caused by a relative of his.

II. The next level was one of simple *causality*. At this level, a person must be a necessary cause of an event in order to be held responsible for that event. For example, Fred would be held responsible for the collapse of a chair that he sat on, even if he could not have foreseen and did not intend the collapse.

III. The third level was one of *foreseeability*, characterized by the attribution of responsibility to a person for acts that he caused and could have foreseen, however unintentional the outcome. At this level, for example, Fred would be held responsible for a fire caused by his smoking in bed, because the outcome of Fred's smoking would be considered foreseeable by the average person.

IV. The fourth level was that of *intention*. Here, an individual would be held responsible only for all intentional acts that he performs. For example, Fred would be held responsible for shooting his hunting partner if and only if he actually intended to injure that person when he pulled the trigger.

V. The final level was that of *justification* based on the criterion of noncoercive environment. For example, Fred should be held responsible for writing a ransom note only if he is not forced into it by a kidnapper (e.g., having a gun pointed at his head while he is writing a ransom note). Similarly, Fred should not be held responsible for attacking someone carrying food home from the market if he were starving and had no money at the time.

It should be noted that according to the distinctions made between causality and responsibility in chapter 1, only levels III through V would qualify as responsibility attributions made on the basis of dimensions in addition to and separate from judgments of causality. It also should be noted that the concept of blame, as defined by Shaver (1985), is not included in Heider's levels given that it involves a later part of a sequential process that only begins with judgments of causality and responsibility.

Heider compared Piaget's distinction between objective and subjective judgments to his own distinction between attributed responsibility at levels II and IV (Shaver, 1985). If one thinks of Heider's stages as descriptions of a developmental progression (a concept that has been critiqued by Shaver, 1985), it can be noted that Heider and Piaget roughly agreed on the direction followed by moral development, although Heider took a more refined and broader view of the possible stages involved. In the subsequent section we will review data addressing the broad conception provided by Heider's developmental perspective.

Testing Heider's Theory of Attributional Development

The first major attempts to test Heider's developmental theory came from studies by Shaw and colleagues. The most noteworthy experiment, conducted by Shaw and Sulzer (1964), compared the responses of children and adults to situations that incorporated different causal dimensions (e.g., intentionality, foreseeability, justification). Stories of interpersonal events involving a person named Perry were presented verbally to two groups of subjects (second graders aged 6 to 9 and college students aged 19 to 38). Each story described an event containing the minimum attributes necessary for determining responsibility at one of the five levels described above. For instance, a level II story involved an unforeseeable accident by Perry, while a level III story involved a foreseeable accident. The corresponding level IV story involved a similar, but intentional (nonaccidental), act by Perry. Each subject heard two stories appropriate to each level, and for each story subjects were asked to rate Perry's degree of responsibility for the event's outcome.

Shaw and Sulzer's assumption was that a particular subject would attribute the most responsibility to Perry in the stories containing characteristics appropriate for the subject's level of attributional sophistication. For example, if college students based their attributions largely on intentionality (level IV), they would be expected to attribute the greatest amount of responsibility to Perry in level IV and V stories. Similarly, second graders, assumed by Piaget to attribute at level II, would attribute responsibility more or less equally in stories at all levels since all stories satisfied the level II criterion of simple causality.

Shaw and Sulzer (1964) found some evidence in support of their hypotheses. They reported a significant interaction between the effects of subject population (second graders vs. college students) and level of stimulus story, indicating the possibility of age-related differences in the responses to Heider's levels. Unfortunately, Shaw and Sulzer failed to report separately the comparisons between attributions at each level of stimulus story (Heider's levels I–V) for the two age groups studied. Thus, there was no evidence that the specific patterns of developmental effects as described by Heider were obtained.

In addition, Shaw and Sulzer's selection of subject groups and preparation of stimulus stories resulted in a seriously confounded design. The large difference in age between the two groups of subjects required a demonstration that the stimulus stories were equally comprehended by both groups. Without this demonstration, the possibility existed that the "children" understood all the stories equally poorly, while the "adults" were familiar enough with the vocabulary and instructions to distinguish one story from another. This comprehension explanation, rather than a developmental progression of moral judgments based on Heider's levels, could explain the interaction between the stimulus levels and population found by Shaw and Sulzer.

Shaw and his associates (Shaw, Bristoe, & Garcia-Esteve, 1968; Shaw & Iwawaki, 1972; Shaw & Schneider, 1969) subsequently conducted a number of similar studies. These studies all produced significant interaction effects of subjects' age and the stimulus stories, but again there were no specific comparisons reported between the attributional patterns of one age group versus another. In addition, the stimulus materials used in all of these studies may not have reflected clearly Heider's levels of responsibility. For instance, the theoretical difference between a level III and a level IV story is the intentionality of the target person's behavior. Although the level III and level IV stories in Shaw's work differed in intentionality, they also differed in other respects. One of Shaw's level III stories was:

Perry was taking his little sister to school. She started to step into a busy street but Perry wanted to look in a store window, so he pulled her back. This kept his sister from being hit by a speeding car (Harris, 1981, p. 68).

The equivalent level IV story is:

Perry was fishing when he saw a boy drowning in the river. Perry could not swim, but he fought his way out to the boy and pulled him out (Harris, 1981, p. 69).

Not only did these stories differ in the intentionality of Perry's action, but also in his effort and ability—that is, the level IV action was one in which Perry's extremely high effort compensated for his lack of a relevant ability, while the level III action involved low effort and adequate ability. Because of this confounding, any developmental differences in subjects' responses did not necessarily reflect differences in perceived intentionality.

A second major test of Heider's developmental theory was Harris's (1977) attempt to improve on Shaw's stimulus stories and on their method of presentation. Five videotaped stimulus events were designed to embody Heider's levels. The events all involved the breaking of a chair that was associated with a young girl named Nancy. In the five events, the chair was broken: (I) by someone besides Nancy, (II) by Nancy accidentally, (III) by Nancy involving a noticeably fragile chair, (IV) by Nancy intentionally, and (V) by Nancy at her mother's request. As in Shaw and Sulzer's (1964) study, Harris's subjects were asked to rate Nancy's naughtiness. A unique feature of Harris's study was the use of an exclusively between-subjects design; each subject saw and rated only one stimulus event.

Using groups of subjects from Grades 1, 3, 6, 8, and college students, Harris found a pattern of attributions that strongly supported Heider's developmental hypothesis. As predicted, the groups of more mature attributors showed increased attributions to Nancy as her behavior became more internally caused. By contrast, the groups of less mature attributors showed relatively high, undifferentiated attributions to all stimulus events.

A third major test of Heider's levels was a study conducted by Fincham and Jaspars (1979). This study used children from Grades, 2, 4, 6, and 8 who responded to five different types of stimulus stories by making evaluations of blame (the word blame was used rather than naughtiness). Results showed that in general, younger children differentiated between one or two of Heider's levels, whereas older children and adults responded differently to four of the five stimulus stories. Of most interest, however, was the fact that subjects of all ages distinguished Heider's levels II (an uncoerced, unintentional act) and V (an uncoerced, intentional act). Thus, it appeared that all subjects were able to note the importance of intention when assigning blame. These data were in line with those reviewed above in which children were asked to rate the naughtiness of peers rather than to assign blame (Armsby, 1971; Fincham, 1985a). These patterns suggest that movement from outcome-based to intention-based judgments of responsibility may occur earlier than middle childhood, as predicted by Piaget.

The fact that intention-based attributions occur at a relatively young age was replicated by Fincham (1981). In this study, finger puppets were used to enact stimulus stories and 6- and 7-year-old children subsequently provided judgments of blame. They also were asked specific "yes/no" questions regarding who caused the outcome, whether the outcome could have been foreseen, if the outcome was intended by the actor, and whether some justification existed for the actor's behavior. These latter questions provided more extensive data regarding children's knowledge of Heiderian concepts, and results indicated that even at the ages of 6 and 7, children were able to use their knowledge of causality, foreseeability, intention, and justification when making judgments of blame.

The fact that such young children demonstrated use of these concepts in making responsibility attributions suggests the need to examine moral judgments made by "less sophisticated" individuals in order to examine more thoroughly the appropriateness of the developmental scheme proposed by Heider (1958). If the levels are learned with age, Heider's theory could be investigated more thoroughly by evaluating younger groups of subjects or groups of children with deprived learning experiences. Fincham (1982b) investigated the latter, and found that culturally deprived second and fourth graders showed less use of Heider's criteria than same-aged peers characterized as nondeprived.[1] Culturally deprived children in both age groups relied primarily on principles of association and causality (levels I and II) to determine judgments of blame, suggesting that Heider's levels may indeed be learned in the order described above. However, as Fincham (1982b) suggested, there remains a need to study further the responses of preschool children who are not characterized as culturally deprived.

Concluding Points

The studies designed to investigate Heider's developmental theories, although limited in number, are encouraging in their support of his basic view of development. The research shows a progression of increasingly elaborate attributional sophistication, although young children have been

---

[1] Cultural deprivation was defined by the school attended. Children came from two schools, one of which had been designated by education authorities as an "educational priority" given the deprived environment from which its students came. The other school was considered by authorities to draw pupils from a more adequate environment (Fincham, 1982b).

able in some cases to use what appeared earlier to be rather sophisticated analyses. As with the research investigating Piaget's theory, however, future research on Heider's developmental scheme would benefit from further consideration of the role of responsibility attributions in subsequent social interactions and affective reactions.

The Attribution of Causality

In the studies reviewed so far, children's attributions of responsibility and blame have been the exclusive focus. As Shaver (1985) suggested and as Heider's developmental perspective implied, attributing responsibility and blame for an event presupposes some attempt at attribution of causality. In general, the developmental process associated with causal attribution has been studied in two ways. First, it has been related to Heider's levels hypothesis, the major tests of which were described above (Fincham & Jaspars, 1979; Harris, 1977). Second, there has been work on developmental aspects of Kelley's (1967) attribution theory, although these studies also do not always distinguish clearly between attributions of causality and responsibility. In the subsequent sections, literature addressing both Heider's and Kelley's ideas will be reviewed. Studies were included if they: (a) used developmental populations and (b) investigated patterns of causal attribution within a social context.

Causality and Heider's Levels of Attribution

As described above, Shaw and Sulzer's (1964) test of Heider's theory exclusively elicited subjects' attributions of responsibility (naughtiness). The subsequent major studies (Fincham & Jaspars, 1979; Harris, 1977), however, elicited attributions of causality as well as responsibility. Each child was asked to rate on a scale of increasing causality, "How much was [name of actor] the reason for/cause of the [outcome of the event in question]?"

In both studies, children's causal attributions showed a developmental progression primarily at the lower levels of Heider's typology. Specifically, after stimulus level I there were fewer age-related differences for the measure of causality than for the measure of naughtiness. In Harris's study, most subjects were able to perceive causality at all levels wherein the actor became a necessary cause (levels II–V). By contrast, subjects' criteria for attribution of naughtiness seemed to vary more with age. In other words, children of different ages were better able to agree about attributions of causality than evaluations of moral responsibility, suggesting that the former concept may be easier to learn. A roughly similar pattern of results was found by Fincham and Jaspars, with most age groups showing more agreement on causal attributions than on attributions of responsibility.

Complimentary results were reported in Fincham's (1982b) examination of attributional patterns in culturally deprived and nondeprived children (see footnote 1). In the nondeprived group, measures of causality were less variable with age than judgments of blame or naughtiness. This pattern was consistent with that reported by Harris (1977) and Fincham and Jaspars (1979). Culturally deprived children, on the other hand, tended to use the same criteria (differentiation between levels I and II, association and causality) to make judgments of both causality and blame. In other words, deprived children were able to differentiate association from causality— that is, they knew that a peer was not necessarily the cause of any negative outcome with which he was associated (e.g., he was standing nearby when an expensive vase toppled off a table). However, they tended to use these same criteria to assign blame, failing to realize that variables other than causality are important when making moral evaluations. These results suggested that the ability to distinguish causality and blame may be an important part of developmental learning in the realm of responsibility attribution (Fincham, 1982b).

The results of these comparisons of simple causality and moral responsibility suggest that the latter is a more complex concept. Of most relevance to this chapter, this concept is complex enough to show developmental differences, either because the criteria utilized require mature cognitive processes, or because socialization gradually changes children's rules for the evaluation of (already perceived) attributional cues. Fincham's (1982b) results, as well as the position taken by Costanzo and Dix (1983) reviewed earlier, lend some support to this latter position. Of course, the distinction between causality and responsibility may be more significant than the two studies cited here indicate, since it is very difficult to elicit from young children a measure of "how much is (s)he the cause of that event?" apart from the more familiar concept of naughtiness.

Concluding Points

Causal attributions probably follow a developmental scheme similar to that of responsibility attributions. However, they appear to be simpler to learn since age differences in causality judgments are less apparent than age differences in the attribution of responsibility. It is likely that judgments of causality rely less on socialization influences and therefore are learned much earlier in life. It still is not clear, however, precisely what socialization processes are influential in the development of either causality or responsibility attributions, although some work on attributional styles of parents provides some insight in this regard (e.g., Dix & Grusec, 1985).

The Developmental Aspects of Kelley's Theory

The Covariation Principle

As noted in chapter 1, the covariation principle is fundamental to Kelley's (1967) attributional model. The basic tenets of covariation need not be reiterated, but the extent to which children use the types of information described by Kelley (consensus, distinctiveness, and consistency) is of interest here.

In an early paper, DiVitto and McArthur (1978) demonstrated that first graders were able to make some logical use of covariation information. First, third, and sixth graders, and college students were presented with pairs of stories in which an "actor" performed some behavior toward a "target" person. In the stories, levels of consensus, consistency, and distinctiveness information were varied, and subjects were asked to rate the actors and targets along dimensions of "kindness/meaness." Although these dependent measures blurred the causality/responsibility distinction, results showed that the youngest children were able to use only consistency and distinctiveness information when making judgments about the actors in the stories. They were unable to use consensus information in their judgments of the actor, and also were unable to use any covariation information to evaluate the target. Sixth graders, on the other hand, were able to use all sources of information to judge both the actor and the target in an adult-like fashion. Third graders showed a pattern of responses indicating a moderate developmental level. In contrast to the youngest group, third graders were able to use consensus information, but only when making attributions about the target person. DiVitto and McArthur's data suggested a developmental increase in the children's ability to use covariation principles, with consensus information apparently the most difficult to integrate. Also, it seemed that consensus information was utilized first in evaluating targets of some act, whereas distinctiveness and consistency principles were applied earliest to those who performed an act.

Contrasting results were reported by Ruble, Feldman, Higgins, and Karlovac (1979). In their study, children as young as 4 and 5 years old showed an ability to use consensus information. Children aged 4 to 5, 8 to 9, and college students were shown videotaped stimuli of an actor choosing an object from an unseen array while four other actors agreed (high consensus) or disagreed (low consensus) with the choice. All subjects in this study were able to use consensus information when asked to attribute the cause for the choice to the actor (person attribution) or to the object chosen (entity attribution).

The conflicting results in the Ruble et al. (1979) and DiVitto and McArthur (1978) studies can be explained via examination of methodological differences (Fincham, 1983a). First, DiVitto and McArthur asked children to make comparative judgments of "niceness" and "meaness" of actors and targets. Ruble et al., on the other hand, asked subjects to assign causality to the actor or the target object. These two tasks, thus, involve very different judgments, with DiVitto and McArthur asking for moral evaluations and Ruble et al. requesting causal attributions. Second, Ruble et al. presented subjects with videotaped stimuli whereas DiVitto and McArthur presented illustrated stories. As was noted earlier in this chapter, videotaped stimuli sometimes have resulted in more adult-like responses for young children (Shultz & Butkowsky, 1977).

More recent research supported DiVitto and McArthur's claim that consensus is the most difficult covariation information for young children to use (e.g., Dix & Herzberger, 1983; Rholes & Walters, 1982). These studies assessed causal rather than responsibility attributions, and found that children were able to use consensus information when making attributional judgments about a target of some behavior prior to being able to use that information in making a person attribution about the actor of the behavior. Although this actor/target attributional pattern differed from DiVitto and McArthur's data, it was supportive of the notion that consensus information was not used consistently by young children.

Dix and Herzberger (1983) offered a salience explanation for these data. In particular, in DiVitto and McArthur's study, actors in all stories behaved in the same way (e.g., they all offered to share a donut with another child). On the other hand, descriptions of the target persons varied across stories (e.g., the target was a child with whom no one else shared or someone with whom many others shared). The variation in descriptions of targets may have made them more salient aspects of the situation such that what appeared to be "consensus-based" target attributions may have resulted from more automatic, perceptual processes than logical, covariation analyses (see chap. 1 for an analysis of the more general consensus debate).

Dix and Herzberger conducted an experiment that supported their salience notion. Although the youngest group of children in their study (6-year-olds) was unable to use consensus information under any conditions (again these results were in support of DiVitto and McArthur's earlier finding), in other age groups the ability to use consensus information was apparent only under conditions in which the behavior of the actor was salient in comparison to the behavior of others. Dix and Herzberger suggested that under conditions of high consensus (everyone in the story acts similarly), no information was particularly salient to children and thus no compelling attribution could be made. A two-step process was proposed wherein attribution to salient information occurs in a developmental scheme initially and quickly. However, when no particularly salient cause is available, more logical covariation analyses occur as more complex cognitive capacities become available in later childhood and adulthood.

Other work has investigated the developmental use of causal schemata (Kelley, 1972a; see chap. 1) which create expectations about interrelationships among consensus, distinctiveness, and consistency information, and allow an individual to make attributions to person, stimulus, or circumstance when complete covariation information is unavailable. Rholes and Walters (1982) presented incomplete covariation information to subjects and reported that children aged 7 years and above showed an ability to use cues associated with both person and circumstance schemata. If complete information about an actor's behavior across time and situations was not available, or if no information about the behavior of others in a similar situation was provided, children were able to make causal attributions based on knowledge of what relationships between these variables typically occur when the person or circumstance is the cause. The use of a person schema (knowledge of interrelationships when a person is the cause) was apparent even earlier, at ages 5 and 6. Only adults, however, were able to use stimulus-schema cues. One explanation provided for these findings was consistent with the ideas of Dix and Herzberger (1983) reviewed above. Namely, other persons are likely to be more salient aspects of a child's environment than any inanimate environmental stimulus. As a result, thoughts and analyses of others' behavior likely receive more attention at an earlier age, and consequently, children develop and use person schemata prior to those involving circumstance and stimulus attributions.

Concluding Points

Children as young as 4 to 5 years old have demonstrated some ability to use certain types of covariation information to make causal attributions in social situations. However, with increasing age children develop improved abilities to utilize more complex concepts such as explicit consensus information and causal schemata in making attributions of causality. The data to date also suggest the possibility that salience of stimuli may developmentally precede the use of more logical analyses as an important influence on causal judgments.

The Discounting Principle

An important concept in causal attribution theory has been what Kelley (1972b) termed "the discounting principle" (see discussion in chap. 1). The essential features of developmental studies of the discounting principle can be seen in portions of Baldwin and Baldwin's (1970) experiment on children's judgments of kindness. (Again, use of this dependent variable seems a more appropriate measure of blame than causality.) Although this study was not intended as a direct test of the discounting principle (which was not identified explicitly by Kelley until 1972), the data are relevant and deserve brief mention here.

In Baldwin and Baldwin (1970), pairs of illustrated stories were presented to children ranging from kindergarten to college age. Of the stories, one pair contrasted adult-requested with spontaneous gift-giving (a child gives his baby brother a toy), whereas another contrasted the spontaneous lending of a toy wagon with lending that followed a brother's promise of a contingent reward. After exposure to these stories, subjects selected the one story from each pair whose actor seemed more kind; subjects' reasons for their selections then were elicited and analyzed. There were significant differences between kindergarten, second-grade, and fourth-grade groups' use of discounting. In general, discounting increased from kindergarten to college age, with a majority of children not discounting internal causes in the presence of external attributes until approximately the fourth grade.

Since Kelley's explicit identification of the discounting principle (Kelley, 1972b), differences in discounting between groups of children and adults have been studied more directly. For example, Shultz, Butkowsky, Pearce, and Shanfield (1975) developed stories that included an action and either an external or internal cause. Kindergarten, fourth-grade, and eighth-grade subjects were asked to estimate whether a second cause was probably involved in the described event. For example, subjects were given an action such as, "Today Johnny is afraid of a dog," and also the (internal) cause, "Johnny is usually afraid of dogs." The subjects' task was to estimate whether another (e.g., external) cause, "The dog is very large" was likely to be present in the event. Fourth and eighth graders showed significant discounting of both internal and external secondary causes, but the judgments of kindergarten children about a possible secondary cause were unaffected by the prior establishment of a primary cause.[2] It is noteworthy that although this assessment of discounting by Shultz et al. was methodologically quite different from that of Baldwin and Baldwin, the two studies found discounting to become the preferred attributional style at roughly similar ages.

In another study, Smith (1975) asked children to listen to story pairs constructed somewhat differently from those of Baldwin and Baldwin (1970). One story in each pair described a child spontaneously selecting one toy to play with, whereas the complementary story described the same behavior following a reward, order, or obligation to play with the toy in question. Using a variety of measurement techniques, Smith assessed children's judgments of the actor's attitude toward the toy with which he/she played. Consistent with other researchers, Smith found that attributions of fourth graders and college students showed consistent discounting (attributing more toy-liking to the first child), whereas kindergarten children showed essentially none, and second graders showed inconsistent use of this principle.

Although these results were similar to those of experiments already discussed, Smith's methodology did not rule out alternative explanations to an attributional one. As pointed out by Karniol and Ross (1976), present-

---

[2] Shultz et al. also studied the development of other attributional schemas, such as Kelley's (1972b) augmentation principle. They found that the more complex schemas were slower to develop than the (relatively simple) schema of discounting alternate causes.

ing story pairs that differ chiefly by the presence or absence of an additional, external cause may elicit effects based on young children's poor memory. To rule out such a memory-based explanation of the developmental use of discounting, Karniol and Ross (1976) employed both memory aids and checks of subjects' understanding of each stimulus story. When these procedures were coupled with stories of sanctioned and unsanctioned toy play (similar to Smith's), an interesting result was found. Not only did kindergarten subjects not discount internal causes in the presence of external sanction, but they consistently saw external causes as indicative of more internal causality. In other words, when kindergarten children were told about Johnny's spontaneously selecting toy X to play with, and about Gerald's playing with toy X after it was selected for him by his mother, the kindergarten children chose Gerald as the one who "really wanted to play with toy X." Termed the "additive principle" by Karniol and Ross (1976), this effect appears to be replaced by discounting as the child matures (see also Cohen, Gelfand, & Hartmann, 1979).

As Fincham (1983a) suggested, however, it may be a mistake to assume that age-related changes in the use of additive and discounting principles occur as a result of a developmental shift in cognitive capabilities. His contention is based on research demonstrating that the apparent "age shift" from use of an additive rule to use of the discounting principle can be influenced by the content of stimulus materials presented. In particular, variables such as the nature of the reward offered (Cohen, Gelfand, Hartmann, Partlow, Montermayor, & Shigetomi, 1979) and the type of activity described (e.g., play or nonplay) influenced children's use of these principles. Hence, Fincham (1983a) suggested that an important research question concerns exactly what processes are responsible for children's use of the additive rule. It is as yet unclear whether the apparent use of such a rule indicates a perceptual difference, limited cognitive ability, or lack of awareness regarding appropriate use of the principle.

Pryor, Rholes, Ruble, and Kriss (1984) proposed an alternative, salience explanation for young children's use of the additive rule. In their study, 5- to 7-, 8- to 12-, and 15- to 18-year-olds were presented with story pairs in which two male children played with a particular toy under constrained (the child's mother instructed him to do so) or unconstrained (the child chose to play with the toy) conditions. The salience of story characters was manipulated by presenting video images of the child, the mother, or the experimenter along with the verbal presentation of stories, the notion being that visual presentation of a person would enhance salience of the person as a causal attribute. For older children (aged 8 and above), salience had no impact on the discounting of internal causes under constrained conditions. However, salience did have a significant impact on the attributions of the youngest group. These children perceived actors to be less internally motivated when the mother, rather than the child, was made salient.

Concluding Points

Developmental progressions in the use of a discounting principle have occurred fairly consistently in the literature, with younger children demonstrating what appears to be an additive rather than discounting strategy. Also, as with the analysis of the covariation principle discussed above, salience probably is an essential variable to be examined in the discounting activity of young children. It may be that only after a particular developmental stage do more logical principles of causal analysis (i.e., discounting) overrule the impact of salient information.

Developing Causal Attribution to Self: The Overjustification effect

The overjustification effect, stated simply, is an application of Kelley's discounting principle to one's self. Suppose, for example, that a child engages in two equally pleasant leisure activities such as checkers and dominoes. If the child receives an external reward for playing dominoes but not for playing checkers, the overjustification effect would predict an eventual reduction in the child's perceived liking of dominoes compared with checkers. In attributional terms, the child's explanation of the event "playing with dominoes" begins to discount "liking dominoes" as a cause because the external reward for playing dominoes becomes a plausible alternative explanation.

Studies of the overjustification effect have found consistent behavioral evidence for its operation with children as young as kindergarten age. In particular, children have shown reduced play with a previously interesting toy after they were rewarded for playing with it (e.g., Greene & Lepper, 1974; Lepper, Greene, & Nisbett, 1983; Ross, 1975). Although this is not an unexpected phenomenon, it does raise the question of why kindergarten-age children show overjustification in their self-attributions but not discounting in their attributions to others.

Explanations of the apparent overjustification/discounting paradox (self/other discrepancy) have included both methodological and theoretical issues. With regard to methodological concerns, at least two hypotheses have been proposed: (a) Overjustification effects may occur at a young age because one's own behavior is perceived as more "real" than the behavior of others (e.g., Shultz & Butkowsky, 1977). Wells and Shultz (1980) tested this hypothesis using preschool subjects, however, and found no differences in overjustification effects noted under "real" and "hypothetical" conditions. (b) In general, studies that reported the overjustification effect in preschool children utilized subjects' behavior (e.g., reduced play with a toy) as a primary dependent variable. On the other hand, studies demonstrating that preschool children were unable to use the discounting principle assessed subjects' judgments about other children rather than their behavior toward specified targets. Consequently, children may learn to make use of the discounting principle with regard to their own actions before they are able to utilize the principle in a judgmental realm.

Wells and Shultz (1980) provided data to support this notion. Preschool children (age 4.3 to 5.4 years) demonstrated a behavioral preference for a previously unrewarded toy during a postexperimental free play period. They did not, however, report a similar preference when asked to rank a group of toys and to predict their own behavior during the upcoming free play period. In other words, children acted out an overjustification effect (became less interested in a previously preferred toy), but were unable to verbalize the proposed explanation for this effect.

With regard to theoretical explanations for the apparent overjustification/discounting paradox, Guttentag and Longfellow (1978) asserted that overjustification depends on an overattention to environmental causes at the expense of internal ones. Considering this statement along with Jones and Nisbett's (1972) proposal of actor/observer differences (see chap. 2), these authors explained that young children's discounting in self-directed attribution (overjustification effect) may be accentuated by their perspective as actors—that is, as actors they attend more closely to external than internal cues. At the same time, their role as observers in other-directed attribution inhibits their discounting of external cues given the focus on internal variables typical of an observer perspective. In other words, young *actors'* attributional perspectives make them insensitive to motives in the face of external cues (overjustification). Young *observers'* overestimation of internal causes retards their development of a discounting tendency.

A second theoretical explanation for the discrepancy in the overjustification and discounting literature was proposed by Kassin and Lepper (1984). These authors proposed a social-developmental analysis, asserting that a child's ability to utilize discounting principles is based on an interaction between age, or developmental level, and specific learning experiences. This model proposed that age interacts with both situational variables to produce apparent use or failure to use discounting. According to the model, a child first should demonstrate discounting-related behavior. At a later developmental stage he/she will demonstrate the ability to make discounting-related judgments, and still later will be able to explain the discounting reasoning behind their judgments and behavior. As noted earlier, Wells and Shultz (1980) verified that discounting-related behavior appears earlier than judgments based on the discounting principle. Similarly, Lepper, Sagotsky, Dafoe, and Greene (1982) reported evidence that children were able to make discounting-related judgments earlier than they were able to explain any of the principles underlying their choices. These data provide some support for the importance of developmental stages in the use of discounting and suggest an explanation for the overjustification/discounting discrepancy related to the methodological critique raised above regarding variations in dependent measures.

A second tenet of Kassin and Lepper's (1984) model maintained that children first demonstrate use of discounting in concrete, familiar situations. Over time, with repeated experience and a minimal level of cognitive competence, they generalize their experiences and develop an abstract notion of discounting that can be applied in novel, unfamiliar social contexts. In support of this idea, Lepper et al. (1982) reported that preschool children were able to use discounting when judging another child's behavior in a very familiar context. Specifically, subjects (with mean age of 4 years, 5 months) were asked about the food preferences of another child who was required to eat one food in order to get a second food. (Food types were bogus and unfamiliar to subjects in order to control for the subjects' own preferences, but in general the scenario was a familiar one.) Subjects' use of discounting was apparent in their judgments that other children would prefer the food that was an "end" to the one that served as a "means" to the end. Children in this condition also were able to verbalize the reasons for their preferences, and explanations appeared consistent with knowledge of the discounting principle. However, in a less familiar "means/end" context (e.g., earning the right to do art activity X following participation in art activity Y), preference for the "end" activity was only marginally significant. Also, in this context, children were unable to provide explanations for their choices. Hence, Lepper et al. (1982) concluded that abstract knowledge of discounting is preceded by the ability to use the principle in specific, familiar contexts. This model may help explain the overjustification/discounting discrepancy since in vivo experience with situations (in which one must make self-attributions) likely leads to more familiarity with a particular context (and therefore more use of the overjustification principle) than vicarious or observational experience in which one makes other-attributions.

Concluding Points

Although young children fail to use the discounting principle when making judgments about the causes of others' behavior, they exhibit use of a similar, overjustification principle in their own actions at a young age. As they grow older, children develop the ability (probably through some interaction of developmental stage and social experience) to make judgments in line with an overjustification principle and to make judgments about others that take into account a discounting analysis.

Future research in this area could benefit from further examination of the specific socialization influences that contribute to development of attributional patterns such as overjustification and discounting. Lepper (1983a) has made some suggestions about other variables that may influence the overjustification effect. These include, but are not limited to, the child's mood and/or temperament and the attractiveness of the toy or activity that is rewarded. Future research also should address more thoroughly the role that these patterns play in subsequent social interactions and affective response. For example, once a child has exhibited an overjustification-based behavior (change in preference for some activity once it has been reinforced), are his/her attitudes and values changed in any way? Does affect change? Are the child's interactions with peers or authority figures (parents, teachers) influenced by the ability to utilize overjustification or discounting principles? (See Lepper, 1983b, for an examination of some of these issues as they might apply within an educational setting.)

From Causality to Responsibility Attributions

Although Heider's proposed levels of responsibility attribution imply a hierarchical movement from judgments of cause to judgments of responsibility, such movement applies to levels of developmental sophistication, not to progression from one type of judgment to another within a single individual. As reviewed much earlier in this chapter, Shaver (1985) has described a theoretical conception of blame assignment that addresses the relationship between causality, responsibility, and blame within a single individual's attributional processing of a single event. A model discussed by Fincham and Shultz (1981) and Shultz and Schleifer (1983), known as the "entailment model," describes a similar process, suggesting that judgments of punishment (probably reflective of blame) entail both judgments of responsibility and causation. Fincham and Shultz (1981) provided support for this model with a sample of adult subjects. Namely, adults' judgments of causation determined responsibility which, in turn, determined restitution decisions (blame). A second study with adult subjects also supported the entailment model (Fincham & Roberts, 1985).

Developmental aspects of the entailment model were examined by Shultz et al. (1986). In their study, children aged 5, 7, 9, and 11 were asked to imagine scenarios in which they had been victimized by another child of the same gender (e.g., the subject's model airplane had been damaged by a peer). In addition to making judgments of causation, responsibility, and restitution for the scenarios, children were asked to sequence the following events: (a) finding out who caused the harm, (b) discovering if the damage was the perpetrator's fault, and (c) requesting restitution for the damage. Results indicated that children 7 years old and greater sequenced the events in the order predicted by the entailment model; that is, judgments of causation preceded judgments of responsibility which, in turn, preceded restitution decisions. Children 5 years old, however, showed a tendency to place restitution first in the sequence. Shultz et al. (1986) suggested that 5-year-olds may have been overconcerned with obtaining restitution, but their data affirmed that these children did not show an inability to understand the concepts of causation or responsibility.

Concluding Points

Developmental investigation of the entailment model and, likewise, the model proposed by Shaver (1985) are avenues worthy of future research. Within this work, it would be useful to investigate children's responses to more complex, "real life" social interactions than those traditionally studied. In the literature reviewed above, children perceived events in which an act and an outcome occurred in close temporal proximity, usually also within the context of a laboratory analogue situation. In the "real world," many more complex behavioral sequences occur, and research with adults has begun to investigate these more complex causal sequences. For example, the phenomenon of intervening causation, or the impact on responsibility attributions of an independent act that occurs temporally between an actor's behavior and a harmful consequence (e.g., Fincham & Roberts, 1985; Fincham & Shultz, 1981; Shultz, Schleifer, & Altman, 1981) has been studied. To the authors' knowledge, however, children's reactions to scenarios involving intervening causes have not been assessed. It certainly would be helpful to know something about the developmental aspects of this phenomenon.

General Concluding Comments

The basic, theoretical work that has been the focus of much of the developmental attribution literature has contributed significantly to our understanding of basic attributional processes. The developmental literature by far has provided the largest body of work addressing conceptual distinctions between causality and responsibility, and in general has provided a framework for the analysis of moral evaluation in subjects of all ages.

Future research on the developmental aspects of responsibility attribution appears to be headed toward a broadening and expansion of early work based on Piaget's and Heider's theoretical perspectives. Of continued interest should be consideration of the relationships among causation, responsibility, and blame assignment, examination of responsibility attributions in more complex social situations, identification of socialization processes that aid development of attribution patterns, and examination of the effects that attribution of responsibility has on subsequent social interactions and affective reactions.

Although developmental attribution research typically has emphasized basic, theoretical research, more applied projects soon should begin to emerge from this work. As the reader will see from subsequent chapters, attribution theory has been applied widely to various aspects of life experience—education, close relationships, health, victimization, and numerous psychiatric or psychological difficulties. To our knowledge, little work within these applied domains has included a developmental perspective. Such a perspective might tell us more about how children learn special attributional rules that apply to situations such as forming friendships, loss of loved ones, and physical or psychiatric illness in oneself, family, or friends. More applied developmental attribution work in these and other realms would serve a transitional role between the more basic, theoretical work described here and the more applied (although not atheoretical) work discussed in subsequent chapters.

Part II Applications

Attributional analyses assume that people are motivated to develop organized, meaningful accounts of the numerous events they observe every day. People are seen as having a need to explain, predict, and try to control their social environments. The attribution of events to invariances and dispositional properties helps to serve this need. This assumption that individuals are motivated to predict and control their environments is central to each of the chapters in this section.

In the first chapter of this part on applications of attributional analyses, we examine the role of attributional processes in close relationships. A central theme of much of this work is that attributions occur frequently in the context of close relationships and serve the purpose of understanding or controlling various aspects of the relationship. Indeed, research suggests that attributional activity often is important to the maintenance, quality, and dissolution of close relationships.

In recent years, increasing attention has been given to the importance of social psychological processes in the prevention, treatment, and maintenance of health-related behavior. In chapter 6, we review research suggesting that causal and responsibility attributions play a role in psychological adjustment to disease, physical disability, sexual assault, and other forms of victimization. One conclusion derived from the attribution-health literature is that explanations for traumatic events that provide individuals with a sense of control over future outcomes probably lead to improved coping.

In chapter 7, we focus not on reactions to traumatic events such as physical disease, disability, or victimization, but more on the role of attributional processes in coping psychologically with everyday problems in living. We examine a number of clinically relevant target behaviors. Specifically, we discuss attributional processes as they relate to Seligman's (e.g., Abramson et al., 1978) learned helplessness model of depression and the relationship of this model to other problems in living, such as loneliness and social anxiety. We also review Storms and McCaul's (1976) model of the emotional exacerbation of dysfunctional behaviors. Finally, we examine research indicating that individuals may employ their psychological symptoms as self-handicapping strategies.

Our discussion of attributional activity as it relates to various dysfunctional behaviors is extended in chapter 8 to focus on the role of attributional processes in the treatment of such behaviors. We examine research relevant to two major forms of attriubtional treatments of maladaptive behavior patterns: misattribution and reattribution-training therapies. In addition, we present evidence suggesting that individuals are more likely to maintain treatment improvements if they assume responsibility for their behavioral changes.

Attribution theory and research has enjoyed widespread application to achievement behavior within educational settings. Students' perceptions of their performance outcomes, along with their analyses of why they succeeded or failed, can have a signficant impact on expectancies for future performance, mood, and subsequent academic behavior. The last chapter of this part reviews theory and research concerned with the achievement–attribution relationship.

5
Attributional Processes in Close Relationships

Introduction

In general, the topic of close, intimate relationships has become a focus for increased theoretical analysis and research in the field of psychology only in the last 15 years. (Clark & Reis, 1988; Kelley et al., 1983). Perhaps it is not surprising, then, that the study of attributional processes in close relationships has emerged also only in the last 15 years. It seems obvious, however, that relationship phenomena have become a major subject for attribution scholars in the 1980s and one that will be pursued vigorously well into the next century. Central to the close relationship is a great amount of interpretive activity on the part of both persons. "Why did he say that—to hurt me?" "What kind of a fool does she think I am; what kind of a game is she playing, anyway?" "He is so sensitive, and I need him so much in my life." "She is the jewel of my life."

These statements are the kinds of common responses that reflect both explicit and implicit attributions made in close relationships. Presumably, they are made to achieve a better understanding of and control over aspects and events of this integral part of people's lives. They are made in the context of different motives and circumstances and reflect a variety of cognitive and emotional processes. Sometimes people form their attributions in relationships only after great deliberation and weighing of evidence (a la the "ANOVA analyst" depicted by Kelley, 1967). At other times, they attribute much more quickly and with less explicit deliberation (not unlike the activity Kelley, 1972a, posited for the operation of causal schemata). Moreover, we find a considerable amount of dispositional imputation in examining people's attributions about their close relationships (cf. Jones & Davis, 1965). Presumably, these attributions get translated directly into behavioral patterns (Yarkin, Harvey, & Bloxom, 1981), or they may be filtered only indirectly into interaction patterns.

One focus in this chapter will be on the relationship between attribution and other cognitive and affective responses in individuals involved in close relationships. While this line of work has been fertile, it should be noted at the outset that the attribution concept also has been found to be useful in other work with relationship implications. For example, Frieze (1979) has studied the attributional processes of battered women. Janoff-Bulman (1978) has studied these processes among rape victims. Shields and Han-neke (1983) have studied the attributions of violent husbands and their wives.

Before we go further in discussing theory and research on attributions and relationships, a definition of a close relationship is in order. Kelley et al. (1983) provide one possible definition of a close relationship as a rela-tionship between two people that is "one of strong, frequent, and diverse interdependence that lasts over a considerable period of time" (p. 38). Kelley and his colleagues go on to define interdependence as a state in which lives are closely intertwined: "The two are tightly bound together by virtue of many strong causal connections between them" (p. 39). While this definition of a close relationship is just one among many, it provides a foundation for our treatment of the attribution–close relationship linkage. We are discussing the more substantial, long-term relationships that people have—not "flings" or relationships that involve little overall time or mutual involvements. Further, most of the work in this area so far has been concerned with heterosexual intimate relationships; little if any work has been done on attribution and same-sex romantic associations or on attribu-tions in various other kinds of bondings such as in familial relations.

Are attribution theorists discovering totally new phenomena in their movement to study relationships? No. Although this line of work on attribution–close relationships is little more than a decade old, it was pre-saged by earlier research done by clinical marriage scholars that pointed to the importance of distortion in distressed spouses' perceptions of self and other (Laing, Phillipson, & Lee, 1966; Murstein & Beck, 1972; Tharp, 1963). Also, communications–family theorists (e.g., Watzlawick, Beavin, & Jackson, 1967) long have held the view that metacommunication be-tween couples (i.e., the implicit meanings conveyed via their interaction) represents a critical factor in determining relationship outcome. The semi-nal study by Raush, Barry, Hertel, and Swain (1974) addressed not only communications questions pertaining to marital interaction, but this work also probed the schemata held by self and other in influencing interaction.

Communicating Affect and Egocentric Attribution

The earliest explicit work on attribution in close relationships evolved from the work of Kelley and his colleagues. Orvis, Kelley, and Butler (1976) asked individuals in romantic partnerships simply to list examples of be-havior, for self and partner, for which each had a different explanation; this procedure was followed in order to minimize the possibility that the proce-dure would actually contribute to discord or conflict. Orvis et al. obtained data from 41 college-aged couples in a sample containing a mixture of dating, married, and cohabiting partnerships. In the questionnaire, individuals not only listed examples of differently explained behaviors, but also provided their own explanations and what they felt would be their partners' explanations of these instances. Respondents' descriptions suggested several categories of behaviors that were explained differently by both partners. Examples of these categories included: Actor criticizes or places demands upon the partner; actor is too involved in outside relationships and activities; and actor inconveniences others. These were not attributions about conflict, per se, by partners contemplating separation. In admitting their awareness of the discrepancies between own and other's accounts of the same actions, the respondents may have indicated a sort of "running attribution" through the course of a relationship from its outset. Awareness of discrepancy at one point may provide the seed for later major attributional conflict.

Orvis et al. (1976) suggested that partners in such close relationships may analyze causality in a manner qualitatively diffeent from that of other actor–observer attributions. In their formulation of the divergent-perspectives hypothesis, Jones and Nisbett (1972) emphasized that actors and observers have different information and thus infer different causes for the same behavior. In the romantic relationships surveyed by Orvis et al., it was found that attributions were colored by intention and anticipation, as well as by different information. Orvis et al. theorized that when partners disagree about the causes of the other's actions, the threat of conflict precipitates an intense and searching causal analysis. The question, "Why did he/she do that?" is embedded among the questions "What can *I* do about this?" and "What *should* he/she do?" As Orvis et al. concluded, in continuing as well as initiating or dissolving close relationships, attribution represents a process of ongoing evaluation and restructuring, whose quality must change as the relationship's basic premises are intensified or altered. The search for causes is undertaken at various times to smooth out the rough spots, identify central issues, and justify the behavior of self or other. A most important aspect of Orvis et al.'s argument is that people in close relationships use attributions to communicate feelings about the relationship. For example, when a person publicly attributes certain relationship problems to a partner's immaturity, the person may be expressing a personal feeling or a desire that the partner change various lines of conduct reflecting on maturity (see Newman, 1981, for a full discussion of the attribution-as-communication thesis).

The Orvis et al. study was the first in a series of investigations that found evidence suggesting a strong dispositional attributional tendency in couples. Further, pejorative trait attributions were found to characterize an individual's attributions for a partner's alleged misdeeds and/or when the couple was experiencing significant distress. A follow-up study by Passer, Kelley, and Michela (1978) was designed to determine the underlying dimensions of attribution reported by subjects in Orvis et al.'s study. This research by Passer et al. produced another important insight, namely: Not only are such couples' attributions often dispositional in nature, but also they frequently implicate dyadic causality (e.g., "His 'momma-boy' tendencies caused us to have problems"). Unfortunately, Passer et al. used a technique that may be low in ecological validity. They asked a sample of college students to respond to a questionnaire while imagining a scene in which members of a couple were involved in a conflict. The questionnaire required them to match 13 attributional categories with scenes worded to reflect either the perspective of the actor (self) or the target of the actor's behavior. The authors then applied a multidimensional scaling procedure to identify the most important attributional categories from both actor and observer perspectives. Based on the dimensions isolated, the authors concluded that subjects perceived actors as concerned with justification and rationalization of negative behavior, while they perceived observers as concerned with how characterological a behavior was.

An egocentric or self-serving bias motive also has been argued by other investigators. In a study by Ross and Sicoly (1979), married coupled were asked to estimate the extent of their responsibility for each of 20 relationship activities by marking a line with end points labeled *primarily wife* and *primarily husband.* The items included making breakfast, cleaning dishes, caring for children, planning leisure activities, making important decisions, causing arguments, making the house messy, and irritating the spouse. Analyses revealed a significant bias; that is, spouses tended to overestimate consistently their own responsibility for relationship events. The authors suggested that the egocentric bias is mediated by selective recall for one's own behavior, since the tendency to recall self-relevant behaviors was highly correlated with overestimation of one's responsibility. This research, however, did not eliminate the possibility that this bias may be mediated by self-esteem motivation (see also McFarland & Ross, 1987, for other evidence relevant to a position emphasizing the role of memory in mediating such attributional tendencies).

These findings were replicated by Thompson and Kelley (1981). In addition, there was a small but significant negative correlation between overall evaluation of the relationship and responsibility for positive events. That is, partners in more satisfactory relationships tended to give more credit to their partners for positive events. Because the number of self-instances recalled correlated significantly with a judgment of self-responsibility, the authors argued that the data support an availability or retrieval bias. Additional data supporting an egocentric bias were obtained by Christensen, Sullaway, and King (1983), who were interested in investigating the frequency of partner agreement on a behavioral checklist of couples' behavior. An egocentric bias based on the hypothesis that partners' disagreements, defined as a greater endorsement of "I" items than "spouse" or "partner" items, was found in both a sample of 50 married and a sample of

50 dating couples. Moreover, subjects showed an increased tendency to attribute responsibility for negative items to the partner as the length of the relationship increased. In a study of college dormitory roommates' perceptions of one another, Sillars (1981) found that college student actors tended to attribute more responsibility for negative behaviors to their roommates than to themselves and to indicate that their own contribution to conflict escalations was less than that of their roommates. This was more true of dissatisfied roommate pairs, while more satisfied pairs tended to internalize conflict responsibility. In addition, other-directed blame and perceived stability of conflict were highest when satisfaction with the roommate was lowest.

In another study that bears on the egocentric-attribution question, Madden and Janoff-Bulman (1983) investigated blame, control, and marital satisfaction in middle-aged respondents. They interviewed married women regarding two standard conflict situations and two conflicts from their own relationship. Results suggested that marital satisfaction was negatively associated with blaming one's husband for relationship difficulties and positively associated with perceived personal control over conflicts. Generally, the wife perceived her husband "as the one who determines how negative problems develop in the marriage, and she perceives herself as the major force behind more positive aspects of the relationship, resolving or entirely avoiding conflicts" (p. 670). Ten of the 15 women who blamed their husbands most were among the least satisfied in the sample: "Of these 10 women, nine specifically mentioned negative personality characteristics of their husbands as a source of their own marital conflicts" (p. 671). Thus, while husbands were perceived as controlling the recurrence and negativity of relationship problems, these wives' tendencies toward characterological blame implied that conflicts would be relatively permanent and unchanging. This evidence is complemented by data obtained by Doherty (1982) in a study of newlyweds' attributions. For hypothetical situations, wives' tendency to infer negative traits on the part of the story character was positively related with self-reported angry responses to statements made by their own spouses.

A final study of discussion in this early vein of work was conducted by Harvey, Wells, and Alvarez (1978). Harvey et al. (1978) examined the ways in which people account for the experience and sources of admitted conflict. Harvey et al. invited participation from couples who had been essentially living together for at least 6 months, and who acknowledged having experienced conflict in their relationship. Harvey et al. asked individuals to judge their own and their partners' perceptions of sources of real conflict and found these attributions to be discrepant. Partners did not agree about the sources of conflict, yet they perceived themselves to be in agreement. One partner assigned a certain weight to a conflict category (e.g., incompatibility in sexual relations) and indicated that the other would give it a similar weight. Although partners in fact did not agree on these issues, apparently they thought that they did agree. Harvey et al. speculated that it is not the agreement of partners that mediates relationships' endurance or breakdown, but rather the perception of agreement between partners. When encountering conflict in close relationships, people may focus their attributional efforts more on the illusion of agreement than on an incisive analysis of the conflict itself.

This evidence suggests that attribution is an ongoing, dynamic activity throughout the course of close relationships. The dynamism comes from the fact that the quality of the attributions must change as the relationship itself intensifies, falters, or terminates. A second study reported in Harvey et al. (1978) indicated that even once the relationship has been terminated, individuals continue to engage in causal analysis. At this stage, however, rather than contributing to relationship "maintenance" or "quality," the attributional queries are part of individuals' self-assessments and rationalizations for the dissolution. In a survey over a 6-month period of separated individuals (mostly women), Harvey et al. found that respondents continued to rehash and ruminate on the whys and wherefores of relationship conflict long after the relationship had ended. These postseparation attributions seemed to focus on fixing blame and adjusting (generally lowering) evaluations of the other and other's significance to the attributing partner (see the discussion below of account-making). Harvey et al. (1978) suggested that attributional analysis may lag behind critical behavior as a relationship moves from conflict to separation. It is possible that partners are busy "being in conflict" and do not afford themselves the luxury of causal analysis (see discussion of Haltzworth-Munroe and Jacobson, 1985, pp. 101–102).

To summarize, there is evidence that people in intimate relationships are biased in the way they apportion responsibility and blame. People tend to take credit for positive relationship events, a phenomenon that may have something to do with selective recall, although the possibility that such a bias is mediated by motivational concerns has not been ruled out. Especially in distressed relationships, a number of studies also indicate that people are likely to blame their partners for negative events. Further, as couples encounter serious conflict, they may become less knowledgeable about how their partners understand the sources of the conflict. They may think they know how their partners think, but they may be badly mistaken. Most of this evidence is correlational in nature and does not indicate causal direction.

Attribution and Depression

The foregoing work is relevant to the general question of attributional style exhibited in close relationships (i.e., the trait variable measured by the Attribution Style Questionnaire, Peterson et al., 1982). The only modicum of explicit evidence pertains to the attribution–depression linkage. Fincham and colleagues have investigated this linkage as a possible mediator of relationship satisfaction (e.g., Fincham & Beach, in press). They found that, as might be expected, depressed mood and marital satisfaction were inversely related. However, using regression analyses, depression was not found to be a significant predictor of satisfaction when entered into a regression equation with the attribution indices employed. On the other hand, attribution of responsibility for positively and negatively valenced relationship events was found to be a significant predictor of relationship satisfaction. No doubt a degree of depression and other major, chronic psychological states may influence the role of attribution in relationship satisfaction. The nature of these associations particularly deserves attention by attribution scholars concerned with clinical aspects of close relationships.

Account-Making

Weiss (1975), a sociologist, conducted a very informative study of marital separation that speaks to the communicative value of attributional accounts about why a close relationship ended. He conducted in-depth interviews with separated persons living in the Boston area. Most of the respondents had been separated for a relatively brief period of time (less than 10 months was the limit in most cases). The data were essentially case-history reports. Both males and females were interviewed, but no attempt was made to compare responses of ex-partners; participants came mainly from the organization called Parents Without Partners. In this work, Weiss essentially introduced the concept of the attributional account to the literature on the psychology of close relationships. The concept in recent years has been increasingly attracting the attention of relationship scholars (see Burnett, McGhee, & Clarke, 1987). In later work on accounts and account-making regarding relationships, accounts have been defined as people's story-like explanations for past actions and events which include characterizations of self and significant others. They are meanings organized into a story and thus represent more than collections of disparate attributions (Harvey, Agostinelli, & Weber, 1989).

Weiss (1975) suggested that people involved in the act of separation develop an account of what happened and why:

The account is of major psychological importance to the separated, not only because it settles the issue of who was responsible for what, but also because it imposes on the confused marital events that preceded the separation a plot structure with a beginning, middle, and end and so organizes the events into a conceptually manageable unity. Once understood in this way, the events can be dealt with (pp. 13–14).

In further discussion of the accounts that people often develop in the act of separation, Weiss implies that divergent explanations are quite pervasive: "None of the events significant to him appeared in her account, nor were any of the events significant for her included in his account" (p. 15). Weiss noted that these divergent accounts usually are selected by individuals from a bewilderingly complex range of events preceding and surrounding a separation, and he noted that accounts, as well as the perceived and actual events upon which they are based, may constantly be reviewed in an obsessive-like ritual performed by the individual in trying to make sense out of what has happened. The accounts represent themes centering on such matters as infidelity and betrayal, a desire for new things in life, perceived overreactions to activities (such as various degrees of extramarital intimacy), and freedom from constraints imposed by the partner.

An interesting example of an account comes from Brende and Parson's (1985) work on the difficulties experienced by Vietnam veterans when they come back home to the United States. This veteran is speaking about the agony he experienced in discovering that his girlfriend could no longer maintain her relationship with him:

My girlfriend told me she didn't know how to relate to me . . . I had expected things to be the way they were; but they weren't. She said she thought I had been killed in the war, because I stopped writing to her. Honestly, I didn't know how to relate to her now either. I dreaded going to bed with her . . . She also said that I wasn't the loving guy she used to know and love, that something horrible must have happened to me over there to change me so completely. I told her I didn't know what she was talking about. She said the look in my eyes was the look of a deeply terrorized person, with a long-distance stare . . . She also mentioned that my frightened look and pallid complexion, my uptight way of sitting, talking, walking, you name it, my aloofness, and all that, made her too uncomfortable for us to continue our relationship. She said that besides, she had found somebody else anyway. That really hurt me (p. 46).

In several recent writings, Harvey, Weber, and their colleagues (e.g., Harvey et al., 1989; Harvey, Weber, Galvin, Huszti, & Garnick, 1986; Weber, Harvey, & Stanley, 1987) have discussed conditions affecting account-making, their motivations, and their possible relationship to interaction and future planning. Some of the motivations for account-making include: (a) the need to establish a sense of personal control; (b) self-esteem maintenance and enhancement; (c) the need for closure; and (d) the desire to persuade others regarding some aspect of one's life, or regarding principles and morals extracted from accounts of these aspects of one's life (Antaki, 1987). Regarding future plans for relationships, Harvey et al. (1989) report data suggesting that people's plans for future relations often follow closely the themes of their accounts for why past relationships ended. For example, an account emphasizing early movement into sexual activity was related to a plan to go slowly and get to know others better in future relations.

The account-making topic is a rich and central one for pursuit among scholars interested in the links between attribution and relationships. The topic has many tentacles in contemporary research. For example, it relates to the sociologists Soctt and Lyman's (1968) work on people's tendency to make excuses and justifications to bolster their self-esteem in problematic situations. It is an essential element of research on turning points in commitment in relationships (Surra, 1985; Surra, Arizzi, & Asmussen, 1988). The topic also is at least strongly implied in the following lines of work: (a) as discussed in chapter 3, Read's (1987) analysis of how people construct causal scenarios (or develop into story-tellers and story-understanders); (b) Rosenblatt's (1983) research on people's griefwork for lost relationships; (c) Folkes's (1982) research on the reasons people communicate to others for rejecting their date overtures; and (d) Shaver, Schwartz, and colleagues' investigations of emotional prototypes which refer to people's implicit understandings of and beliefs about emotions (e.g., see Schwartz & Shaver, 1987). It should be noted that Surra (1988) has provided a useful coding manual for use with certain kinds of free-response attributions. Also, Fletcher (1983) and Harvey, Turnquist, and Agostinelli (1988) have addressed methodological issues involved in studying various types of free-response attributional activity, including account-making. These issues include the definition and coding of attribution along dimensions such as valence, and whether the attribution reflects internality and/or controllability of perceived locus of causality. Overall, coding issues and the need for greater theoretical development represent major agenda items for future work on the psychology of account-making.

Attributional Differences in Distressed and Nondistressed Couples

Much of the recent work on attributions in close relationships has been done by clinical researchers focusing on the dynamics of marital distress. The typical method has involved solicitation of respondent couples from couples seeking therapy at university clinical facilities. As Fincham and Bradbury (in press) note, we do not have evidence on the possible differences in attributional tendencies among such couples as compared to other couples—including those who do not want to participate in the research.

The often-reported major differences between distressed and nondistressed couples in their negative and positive behavior toward spouses (e.g., Gottman, 1979; Jacobson, Folette, & McDonald, 1982) have led researchers to examine attributions for behaviors that differ in valence. It has been hypothesized and found that distressed couples are more likely to make causal attributions which undermine or neutralize positive spouse behavior but which accentuate the impact of negative behaviors; these attributions then are related to subsequent responses to such behavior (cf. Kelley & Michela, 1980). As an illustrative study in this genre, Jacobson, McDonald, Folette, and Berley (1985) investigated the extent to which distressed spouses attribute positive partner behaviors to external factors while attributing negative behavior to internal factors. Unknown to one spouse, the other was instructed to "act positive" or "act negative" on a conflict resolution task following which the uniformed spouse rated a set of causal attributions for their partner's behavior. Overall, there was a tendency to favor internal attributions, which is consistent with previous research showing that partner behavior is explained in dispositional terms (cf. Kelley, 1979), but differences nonetheless emerged between the two groups. Distressed couples rated negative spouse behavior more internally, whereas nondistressed couples did so for positive spouse behavior.

As Berley and Jacobson (1984) suggest, these results support one of the ideas that was discussed in the previous section. The results suggest an expectancy or consistency effect: Distressed couples, having established negative transactional patterns, attribute expected negative behaviors to dispositional influences. As Heider's (1958) balance theory suggests, we expect good people to perform good actions and bad people to perform bad actions. Spouses in distressed relationships are likely to feel helpless and ineffectual in generating behavior changes in their partners. Negative dispositional attributions ("He's a bastard because of the way he has been treating me") can be used to justify the typical pattern in distressed relationships of escalating coercive exchanges. Consequently, by attributing their partner's negative behavior to internal, enduring characteristics, they justify their feelings of helplessness and enhance their own self-esteem.

In another study that examined differences between distressed and nondistressed married couples in their attributional tendencies, Fincham and O'Leary (1983) presented 16 distressed and 16 nondistressed married couples with an attribution questionnaire consisting of 12 hypothetical situations. The couples were asked to "vividly imagine yourself in the situations" (p. 47). For each situation, subjects were asked to name the major cause for the behavior and then rate the importance of a series of causal dimensions, using Likert scales. The first dimension contrasted causes having to do with a partner with those having to do with external circumstances. The next two dimensions were derived from the categories of Abramson et al. (1978) of *stable–unstable* (referring to the extent to which the cause is likely to be manifested on future occasions) and *global–specific* (reflecting the extent to which the cause is viewed as specific to the behavior as opposed to global). The final dimension was that of *controllable–uncontrollable*, derived from the work of Weiner (1979) on achievement motivation. Subjects were also asked to rate their global affect response to each event on a 7-point scale ranging from *extremely negative* to *extremely positive*. For positive acts, distressed and nondistressed couples differed significantly on the dimensions of globality and controllability. That is, nondistressed spouses saw the causes of positive acts as being more global and more controllable than their distressed counterparts. For negative behaviors, distressed and nondistressed spouses differed only on the dimension of perceived globality, with distressed couples considering the cause to be more global than nondistressed couples. There was also a tendency for distressed couples to rate the cause of negative behavior as more controllable. These results generally were replicated and extended by Fincham, Beach, and Baucom (1987) who examined but found no differences in self-attributions between distressed and nondistressed groups. Also, Kyle and Falbo (1985) found that individuals in distressed marriages tended to explain their spouses' hypothetical negative behavior more dispositionally and their spouses' positive behavior more situationally than did individuals in less distressed marriages. Overall, this line of research deserves further attention within naturalistic contexts of relationship interaction.

The earlier findings of Jacobson et al. (1985) between distressed and nondistressed couples regarding attributional differences have been confirmed and extended in further research by Jacobson and his associates in their fertile program on this topic. An important extension has been reported by Holtzworth-Munroe and Jacobson (1985). In this study, 20 nondistressed and 20 distressed couples listed their thoughts and feelings about partner-initiated behaviors. These behaviors varied in frequency of occurrence and in positive–negative valence. The thought-listing technique employed (the first such study in the attribution–close relationships area) followed the guide of Harvey et al. (1980), who initially reported evidence for a so-called unsolicited attribution method and a related technique reported by Wong and Weiner (1981).

Holtzworth-Munroe and Jacobson (1985) found that husbands in unsatisfying relationships reported more attributional thoughts than did happily married husbands, while wives in the two groups did not differ. Also, behaviors having a negative impact elicited more attributional activity than did positive behaviors. Distressed spouses produced attributional thoughts most often for frequently occurring negative behaviors and produced more attributional thoughts for these events than did their nondistressed counterparts. The attributions also differed in content, with distressed couples producing relatively fewer relationship-enhancing attributions (e.g., "His helping me really showed how much we love one another") and relatively more distress-maintaining attributions (e.g., "His failure to help me is another indication of how things have changed for the worse in our marriage"). Last, the data replicated Fincham and O'Leary's (1983) finding that distressed couples viewed the cause of negative behavior by their spouse as relatively controllable.

Holtzworth-Munroe and Jacobson (1985) advanced the interesting interpretation for their data that as long as positive outcomes obtain, men are lulled into attributional complacency whereas women engage in a degree of attributional activity regardless of level of marital satisfaction. Hence, men rather than women are deemed to be attributional "barometers" of relationship satisfaction. For both men and women, there was a disinclination toward attributional activity for distressed couples following frequent positive partner behaviors. However, for these couples, frequent negative partner behaviors elicited a high degree of attributional activity. As the authors suggest, major distress in the relationship may lead to cognitive fixation on negative behaviors. It seems likely that this tendency is part of the self-fulfilling spiral toward dissolution that couples often encounter (cf. Laing, 1961). Overall, with a relatively nonreactive method, Holtzworth-Munroe and Jacobson's data are consistent with earlier evidence that distressed couples discredit their partners' positive behaviors and maximize cognitive concern with their partners' negative behaviors.

The general topic of assessing spontaneous attributions in marital interaction has been discussed by Bradbury and Fincham (1988). They suggest that such work is subject to a number of questions, including: Does the investigator know the base rate of events for which attributions are being made and the specific content of marital interactions in which attributions occur? Has the investigator conceptually distinguished types of attribution and the functions they play in marital interaction? The investigation of naturalistic attribution in couples promises to be a topic for fruitful inquiry for some time to come.

Cognition in Marriage

In recent years, work on attributions in married couples has been advanced considerably by the research program being carried out by Fincham and colleagues. The general objective of this program is to develop a conceptual understanding of cognition in marriage, with attribution representing a prominent type of such cognition (see Fincham & Bradbury, in press). In addition to the research described above, other work has focused on following relationships over a period of time to probe possible change in attribution. For example, Fletcher, Fincham, Cramer, and Heron (1987) reported that for dating couples attributional activity was greatest early in the relationship and that couples who were most satisfied attributed more equal causal inputs to the relationship. In another study, Fincham and Bradbury (1987) studied 34 couples over 12 months and found that wives' marital satisfaction in particular is related to causal and responsibility attributions for hypothetical spouse behaviors. In general, Fincham (1985b) has proposed that the very occurrence of attribution may be the critical factor in distinguishing distressed versus nondistressed couples. Such a position now at least has as its foundation evidence from many studies across different laboratories and investigators. Whether attribution is *the* critical factor relative to *a* critical factor, however, remains to be determined.

Fincham and his colleagues are most persuasive in arguing that responsibility rather than causality attributions are most common in the different attribution patterns of distressed and nondistressed couples. They also have begun to make a good case that attributions play a causal role in influencing marital satisfaction and that this role is not offset by "third variables" such as depression or prior relationship satisfaction. Fincham and his associates now have begun to try to assess the relationship between attributions and marital behavior. The work thus far is promising but far from conclusive. As Fincham and Bradbury (in press) suggest, it is important to show that an attribution for a specific partner behavior is related to the spouse's subsequent behavior toward the partner. Clearly, one of the most important steps taken by these investigators to date is their examination of attributions in relationships using longitudinal designs.

Attribution Therapy with Couples

A topic to mention briefly here concerns Jacobson and colleagues' (see Berley & Jacobson, 1984) success in using attributional ideas with distressed couples. While embryonic in nature and scope, this work has shown good results with techniques that involve challenging couples' attributions ("Are you sure you've carefully analyzed why she is moody?") and relabeling couples' attributions ("It sounds like she really is trying hard to please you rather than trying to use you"), and behavioral enactment (involving role-playing, rehearsal as well as attributional interventions.). The merit of this collage of attributional approaches to therapy requires further examination by other scholar-clinicians. It appears to have great promise.

Attributions about Commitment in Premarital Relationships

A final set of recent studies deserves mention because of its increasing prominence and focus on attribution in close relationships. This work is being conducted by Huston and his colleagues, and it focuses on attributions made about significant changes in involvement level during the course of a premarital courtship. The method employed in these studies is called the "retrospective interview technique" (Fitzgerald & Surra, 1981). It involves asking respondents to construct a relationship trajectory on a "change of marriage" graph with a 0 to 100% scale. The trajectory or curve serves as a pictorial representation of the relationship in terms of how gradually or rapidly the couple became involved, the level of commitment reached by the couple, the number of ups and downs that occurred, and the rate of dissolution of the relationship.

Studies using this technique and reporting attribution data have been conducted by Lloyd and Cate (1985), Surra (1985), Cate, Huston, and Nesselroade (1986), and Surra et al. (1988). Illustrative findings from this work are the following: Cate et al. (1986) identified a set of types of curves typical of progress toward commitment. For example, a slow rocky (conflict-ridden accent of involvement) was one such type of curve. Surra (1978) in turn found that regardless of type of curve a great percentage of the young persons made dyadic attributions for turning points toward or away from greater commitment. An interesting example she identified was ". . . that was when I told him I had been a prostitute, and he said he still loved me" (p. 51). But Lloyd and Cate's (1985) data indicate that as a breakup starts to occur, individual (or nondyadic) attributions predominate.

Summary and Conclusions

This topic of attribution and close relationships emerged only in the last decade or so but already reflects a fertile area for contemporary attribution work. Early work revealed the role of attribution in communication of affect in relationships. It also pointed to the pervasiveness of egocentric attribution, especially in conflict-oriented relationships. Subsequent work focused on account-making as a key vehicle for coping with the loss of a loved one and with many possible attributional differences between distressed and nondistressed couples. Other work has explored attributions about commitment and the role of memory and attribution in dating partners. A modest amount of work has been done using a type of couples therapy that emphasizes examination of interpretation and advocates challenge of attributions made within distressed couples.

What is the future for this area of work? The area has considerable promise especially as prospective research is done to investigate how couples make attributions during the middle stages, and later in relationships that eventually end. But many questions remain. One interesting query suggested by Antaki (1987) and Fincham and Bradbury (in press) pertains to the "public versus private" nature of the attributions obtained from respondent couples. Most of the work done so far examined private attributions. Yet it seems likely that couples often negotiate attributions and/or develop relationship attributions in discussions with third parties. In such cases, self-presentation dynamics may be heavily involved in the attribution process (see chap. 2). To date, most of the research in this area has been done with cross-sectional retrospective designs. In this regard, the work of Surra and colleagues (e.g., Surra et al., 1988) is promising in its delineation of the reasons people give in making commitments and then how those reasons are related to relationship turning points, including termination. This work involved both cross-sectional and longitudinal design features.

Further inquiry may focus more intensively on archival data. The many sources of archival data available permit the examination of attributions in relationships as in accounts given in diaries. This line of work only has begun to receive the attention it deserves (e.g., Rosenblatt's, 1983, brilliant analysis of 19th-century diaries as evidence about griefwork). More generally, whether in terms of relational process in all couples or of therapy with distressed couples, considerable future work can be fruitfully directed toward probing the rich linkages of thought and action represented by attribution and close relationship interaction patterns. Different types of cross-sectional group designs as well as longitudinal designs can be used to carry out this type of research. Also, different respondent populations must be given more attention. We are an aging society, yet social scientists are only beginning to probe tropics such as close relationships and the elderly (e.g., Matthews, 1986).

The conceptual and methodological issues confronting attribution–relationship research are similar to those facing the burgeoning field of the psychology of close relationships in general (see Clark & Reiss, 1988). The conclusion of our coverage, however, should not stress limitation. Rather, we should emphasize the great promise for discovery in the field and its evolving stature as a scientifically reputable venue of research.

6
Attribution and
Health-Related Functioning

In recent years, probably one of the most burgeoning interfaces within psychology has involved the application of social-psychological theories within the arena of health psychology (Harvey, Bratt, & Lennox, 1987; Spring, Chiodo, & Bowen, 1987). Work in this area has addressed the roles that social-psychological variables and processes play in the prevention, treatment, and maintenance of health-related behavior as well as the functions they serve in psychological adjustment to disease, disability, and other forms of victimization. Research in the social/health domain has focused on numerous topics such as the relationship between psychosocial variables and cancer (Eysenck, 1987; Grossarth-Maticek, Bastiaans, & Kanazir, 1985; Meyerowitz, 1980; Wortman & Dunkel-Schetter, 1979), the effects of stress and stress inoculation on immune functioning (Kiecolt-Glaser et al., 1984; Kiecolt-Glaser, Glaser, et al., 1985), and the influence of psychosocial factors on the adjustment of burn patients (Andreasen, Noyes, & Hartford, 1972).

Within this larger context of a social psychology–health behavior interface, there is a growing body of literature addressing the more specific relationships between attributions and health-related functioning (Michela & Wood, 1986). It is this literature that will be addressed in the present chapter. Various domains of health-related functioning have been linked to attributional processes, and the present chapter will review empirical and theoretical links between attributional activity and coronary-prone behavior, smoking, and victimization in the form of physical injury, sexual assault, and chronic or terminal disease. Although we realize that these areas do not exhaust the available literature, they provide a representative sample of the research questions, hypotheses, methodologies, and issues of interest to attribution research in health psychology. By far the largest volume of work has fallen under the rubric of victimization, and it is with this topic that we begin our discussion.

Victimization

A victim has been defined in the psychological literature as anyone who suffers a change in general life condition as a result of some physical or psychological loss (Janoff-Bulman & Frieze, 1983; Tait & Silver, in press). According to this definition, victims include individuals who have experienced life changes as a result of criminal and/or sexual assualt, natural disaster, chronic or terminal illness, or physically debilitating accidents. Despite the fact that these modes of victimization vary along a number of dimensions (e.g., they can be human-induced or naturally induced, and can occur as a result either of a single, discrete event or a prolonged condition), there appear to be commonalities in the responses exhibited by victims following occurrence of these traumatizing events. For instance, common reactions to victimization include shock, confusion, helplessness, anxiety, and depression (Janoff-Bulman & Frieze, 1983). In addition, victimization can lead to loss of self-esteem, feelings that one has lost control, and aversive or ambivalent reactions from others. Victims of negative life events also can experience a loss of meaning, a need for discussion of the event with others (that at times may be thwarted by social expectations that one portray a coping image), and persistent, intrusive ruminations relative to the event (Tait & Silver, in press).

The severity with which these symptoms can be experienced is attested to by the presence of a discrete diagnostic category in the psychiatric nomenclature (DSM-III-R: American Psychiatric Association 1987) called posttraumatic stress disorder. Individuals who meet criteria for this psychiatric disorder experience as a result of some traumatic event recurrent recollections, flashbacks, and dreams about the event as well as intense distress in the presence of stimuli that evoke memories of the event. They often avoid any situations or feelings associated with the event, and can experience a variety of other psychiatric symptoms such as irritability, difficulty concentrating, estrangement from others, decreased interest in daily living, sleep difficulties, and restricted affect.

Although not all victims experience this set of severely debilitating symptoms, most victims experience some adjustment difficulties. Of particular concern to psychologists interested in victimization is a set of questions including identification of the ways in which victims cope with thier losses, identification of which coping strategies are most adaptive under various conditions of victimization, and theoretical examination of the motives that drive various coping patterns. In line with these questions, three major theories of responses to victimization have been proposed throughout the last 20–25 years. Although these three theories originally dealt with perceptions of a victimized individual held by a nonvictimized party, i.e., an observer, social psychologists more recently have attempted to apply these perspectives to develop an understanding of the victim's own reactions to traumatic events.

The first of these theories, the just-world hypothesis (Lerner, 1965; Lerner & Miller, 1978), proposed that reactions to victimization develop as a result of the need to believe in an orderly, just world wherein people get what they deserve. A second hypothesis, proposed by Shaver (1970), suggested that responses to victimization are designed to protect self-esteem. A third theoretical position (Kelley, 1971; Walster, 1966) stated that reactions to victimization are based on the desire to maintain a belief in control over one's environment. It also is possible that all three of these perspectives could be united under a common theme of desire for control and self-protection. Specifically, the motivation to believe in an orderly world as well as the desire to maintain self-esteem can be thought of as variants of a need to feel protected from or in control of future negative outcomes. Although some of the studies reviewed subsequently attempted to pit these perspectives against one another, the uniqueness of each perspective is not entirely clear.

In consideration of these three perspectives, it should be noted that much of the literature to be reviewed is correlational in nature and therefore does not address directly the causal direction issue. In other words, it is not always clear (even when significant relationships exist) whether attributional patterns are *created* by desire for control, for example, or whether attributions are the *cause* of different adaptational patterns. It also is possible that attributions are simply correlates of certain coping patterns or mood states. In that case, attributions could exist without the presence of any complex mediating variable such as desire for control, belief in a just world, or desire to protect self-esteem (Turnquist, Harvey, & Andersen, 1988).

Despite the correlational nature of the literature, most of the work has focused on the possibility that some kind of motivational state created following a traumatic event drives the search for attributions. In accordance with this perspective, it has been suggested that numerous cognitive assumptions about the world are challenged when an individual is victimized, and that victimization itself initiates a search for ways to restore belief in these assumptions (Janoff-Bulman & Frieze, 1983; Silver, Boon, & Stones, 1983; Tait & Silver, in press). Beliefs in the existence of a controllable, meaningful, and orderly world are contested by victimizing events, often as well as assumptions that one is invulnerable to victimization and in control of one's fate. Janoff-Bulman and Frieze (1983) also suggested that victimization challenges assumptions about one's self-worth. In attempts to explain how victims come to terms with these challenges and restore belief in an orderly and controllable world, an important distinction has been made between attempts to exert primary and secondary control. The former occurs when an individual tries to change the environment to bring it into line with beliefs, whereas secondary control involves a process of adjusting one's "internal structure" to fit a modified environment (Rothbaum, Weisz, & Snyder, 1982). It is the latter type of control that is the basis for the majority of work to be discussed here.

Following victimization, individuals may attempt to gain secondary control and restore belief in an orderly, meaningful world via a variety of cognitive strategies. First, individuals may attempt to *redefine the victimizing experience* in a positive way. For example, parents of children at high risk for developmental disabilities as a result of severe perinatal medical problems reported benefits accruing to themselves and/or their families (e.g., emotional or spiritual growth, improved family relationships) as a result of their infants' physical difficulties (Affleck, Tennen, & Gershman, 1985). In addition, 60% of a sample of breast cancer patients reported the ability to find some beneficial outcomes (such as increased enjoyment of life and improved self-understanding) following diagnosis of their illnesses (Taylor, Wood, & Lichtman, 1983).

Second, victims may attempt to restore control and/or meaning by *minimizing their plights* in a variety of ways. Taylor et al. (1983) reviewed and provided examples of some of these strategies such as: (a) victims at times attempt to compare themselves with others who are "worse off" than they, (b) they sometimes create hypothetical "worse worlds" wherein much more drastic disasters could have occurred had circumstances been different, and (c) some victims manufacture normative standards against which their own adjustment fares well ("I'm doing well under the circumstances").

Third, victims may try to restore assumptions about control and/or a just world via *attributional strategies* designed to assign causality, responsibility, and/or blame in ways that will improve coping. This perspective fits very early notions suggesting that sudden threats or changes in one's environment lead to initiation of a search for causes to enhance understanding of the event (see chap. 1 of this volume; Kelley, 1967; Wong & Weiner, 1981). On the other hand, coping at times may be enhanced by attributional ambiguity, or uncertainty regarding the specific causes of an event (Snyder & Wicklund, 1981). It may be to an individual's advantage, for example, to attribute a traumatic event to a variety of causes in order to protect perceptions of a single cause such as "It was my fault." This aspect of attributional activity has not been addressed explicitly in the victimization literature, but may be of help in understanding why people sometimes invoke multiple causes to explain physical or psychological loss.

In the subsequent sections, we will review empirical findings that relate specific attributional patterns with adjustment following various types of victimization. As will be noted, a primary issue within this literature is the role of self-blame following victimization. As our review will show, there are numerous inconsistencies with regard to this and other issues in the literature. Hence, subsequent to our discussion of relevant empirical findings, we will review methodological and theoretical issues in interpretation of this literature.

Physical Injury

In one of the earliest and most well-known investigations within this literature, Janoff-Bulman and Wortman (1977) interviewed victims of spinal cord injuries resulting from severe, specifiable accidents (rather than birth or disease). All victims were either paraplegic (paralyzed in the lower half of the body) or quadriplegic (paralyzed from the neck down), and had suffered their accidents either 1 to 4 or 8 to 12 months prior to being interviewed. Victims were asked a number of questions in an attempt to characterize their patterns of attribution about the accidents. First, they were asked if they had ever posed to themselves the question, "Why me?," and if so how they had answered it. Second, they were asked to allocate a total of 100% blame for the accident to four factors: self, others, the environment, and chance. Finally, victims were asked to rate the amount of self-blame they felt for the accident and to estimate the degree to which they felt that their accidents had been avoidable. All victims were hospitalized during the evaluation, and nurses and social workers assigned to each patient were asked to rate the degree to which the patient was coping well with his/her disability.

All 29 patients reported that they had asked the question, "Why me?," and all but 1 had come up with at least one possible explanation for the accidents (10 subjects chose to explain their accidents with two hypotheses). Explanations to this open-ended question fell into six categories: (a) predetermination (the accident was predetermined and due to fate), (b) probability (bad things are bound to happen), (c) chance, (d) "God had a reason," (e) deservedness (the accident was deserved due to errors made by the victim), and (f) reevaluation of the event as positive (the accident led to emotional or spiritual growth, increased appreciation of life). The most popular of these explanations was "God had a reason," but none of the explanations presented in this open-ended form was correlated significantly with degree of coping.

Different results emerged, however, when victims rated their attributions with structured measures. First, 62% of the victims attributed *some* degree of blame to themselves and 35% attributed *at least half* of the blame for the accident to themselves (these estimates were based on a single self-blame index that combined victims' responses to the two separate self-blame questions). Second, higher estimates of the victims' coping were made by nurses and social workers when victims reported higher ratings of self-blame, lower ratings of blame assigned to others, and lower estimates of perceived avoidability. In other words, victims were evaluated as coping better if they blamed themselves for the accident, placed little blame on others, and felt they could not have avoided the accident.[1]

---

[1] A much later study by Brewin (1984) also demonstrated a positive relationship between self-blame (defined as a moral evaluation of deservedness) and recovery rate in victims of industrial accidents. However, other data have suggested that

Janoff-Bulman and Wortman (1977) interpreted these data as supporting a just-world hypothesis. Although the majority of the victims clearly stated that they had not "deserved" the accident, the rather high percentage of victims reporting some degree of self-blame (even when the situation did not necessarily warrant such), as well as the relationship between self-blame and coping, were consistent with such an interpretation. Individuals coped better with severe physical disability if they believed that the outcome was due to something about themselves (e.g., I caused my own problems). Under these conditions, the world could be perceived as an orderly place wherein outcomes followed logically and meaningfully from actions. Further support for a just-world interpretation came from results suggesting that coping was poorer when accident outcomes were attributed to other people. In these cases, the world may have been perceived as "unjust"—that is, *I* have a severe disability because of something *you* did—and under these circumstances it may have been more difficult for the patients to cope with such severe outcomes.

Although these data also appear to be consistent with the hypothesis that attributions enhance feelings of control (self-blame enhances feelings of control and thereby improves coping), the relationship between perceived avoidability and coping suggested otherwise. Many victims reported that their accidents had been unavoidable—that is, they had exerted little control over the outcomes—and stronger perceptions of unavoidability were associated with higher estimates of coping. In other words, the greater the belief that the outcome had been unavoidable, the better the victims were rated as coping with their disabilities. These data suggested that exaggerating perceptions of personal control (e.g., I could have avoided that accident) may not have been adaptive when the negative outcome was permanent and nonmodifiable (Janoff-Bulman & Wortman, 1977). However, perceptions of control over future accidents were not measured and it is possible that perceived unavoidability of a past outcome taught the individuals something about how to control future outcomes. If this pattern occurred, control could still be an important moderating variable in the attribution–coping relationship.

In sum, among a sample of 29 spinal-cord-injury patients, those who were rated as coping most effectively were individuals who perceived their accident outcome to be a logical and unavoidable consequence of a freely chosen behavior. However, the precise mechanism through which this relationship occurred was unclear.

In an attempt to understand these relationships more clearly, it was noted that the precise meaning attached by subjects in Janoff-Bulman and Wortman's (1977) sample to perceptions of self-blame was somewhat unclear. Janoff-Bulman (1979) attempted to clarify the concept by making a

---

positive relationships between self-blame and coping may attenuate as significant amounts of time pass following victimization (Schulz & Decker, 1985).

distinction between two types of self-blame: behavioral and characterological. Behavioral blame, or attribution of blame to one's behavior, allows one to perceive that future similar outcomes can be controlled if one merely changes one's behavior. Characterological self-blame, on the other hand, implies that some unmodifiable aspect of personality caused the previous outcomes and may create similar outcomes in the future. In the latter case, self-attribution may interfere with coping. This distinction has been addressed in the majority of work conducted subsequent to the Janoff-Bulman and Wortman (1977) article.

Utilizing the distinction, for example, Kiecolt-Glaser and Williams (1987) examined the relationship between attributional patterns and coping among 49 hospitalized burn patients. The type of accidents resulting in burns included utility and electrical fires, industrial or kitchen accidents, and being set on fire by someone else (in one case the victim set himself on fire). Coping in these patients was rated by each patient's primary nurse and by the physical therapist assigned to work daily with all patients. Measures of coping included evaluations of compliance with medical procedures and ratings of the frequency with which patients mentioned their pain or discomfort. The patients themselves rated the degree to which they attributed blame for their burns to themselves, others, the environment, and chance, and characterized self-blame as being due to behavioral or characterological variables. They also estimated the degree to which they perceived their accidents to have been avoidable, whether they had ever asked themselves the question, "Why me?" and if so, what answers they had chosen as likely hypotheses. Self-report measures of depression and anxiety also were collected.

Results of the Kiecolt-Glaser and Williams (1987) study were somewhat different from those reported by Janoff-Bulman and Wortman (1977). Specifically, over 50% of the sample ($n = 26$) had never asked the question, "Why me?," and an additional 13 patients had asked the question but had found no answer. (Although, of the remaining subjects, "God had a reason" again was one of the most frequent attributions provided.) With regard to the less open-ended questions, over half of the burn patients attributed no blame to themselves for their accidents and only 27% assigned over 50% of the blame to themselves. (These findings were consistent with those of Schulz and Decker, 1985, who found that over 50% of a sample of spinal-cord-injury patients accepted no blame for their injuries.) Within this latter group, the majority of patients indicated that self-blame was of a behavioral nature. Correlational analyses indicated that increased ratings of self-blame (described by subjects as being largely behavioral in nature) were associated with poorer compliance, more frequent mention of pain, and increased levels of depression. These relationships, which contrasted sharply with the results of Janoff-Bulman and Wortman (1977), occurred when both severity of the burn and time since hospital admission were held constant.

Kiecolt-Glaser and Williams (1987) provided a number of explanations for the divergence in results. Possible hypotheses included the following: (a) differences in the pervasiveness with which burn and spinal cord injuries influence life functioning, (b) age of subjects (burn patients were older than the spinal-cord-injury patients), and (c) timing of the interview (burn patients were interviewed within 1 month of their accidents whereas spinal-cord patients were interviewed either 1 to 4 or 8 to 12 months following their accidents). An additional difference suggested by Kiecolt-Glaser and Williams involved possible personality differences between members of the two samples. They reviewed data suggesting that spinal-cord-injury victims often include younger, impulse-dominated men prone to be involved in higher risk activity. Self-blame among these individuals is supposed to be low (Shapiro, 1965), although Janoff-Bulman and Wortman (1977) reported that incidence of self-blame in their sample was rather high. However, it might be that personality style exerts a significant impact on the relationship between self-blame and coping. Such an hypothesis certainly deserves further attention, and will be discussed in more detail below.

Sexual Assault

Victims of sexual assault comprise another population in which the relationship between attributions and coping with victimization has been examined. Within this literature, studies have addressed coping in victims of rape and incest, and speculations have been made with regard to coping in spouse-abuse victims. Although the latter population does not always experience sexual assault, these victims seem more closely aligned with sexual-assault victims than with the other populations discussed in this chapter and therefore will be included here.

Rape Victims

Janoff-Bulman (1979) conducted the first investigation in this area. As noted above, this paper provided an extremely influential thesis regarding the distinction between behavioral and characterological self-blame. Janoff-Bulman proposed that such a distinction could explain differential adjustment patterns associated with self-blame in depressed subjects and rape victims. Self-blame for problems was a common pattern associated with depression, although earlier reports indicated that self-blame in rape victims was associated with more adaptive functioning. Janoff-Bulman (1979) proposed that if self-blame for negative outcomes involved attributions to stable aspects of personality, hopelessness and depression should result since personal control could not be exerted to change personality and thereby modify the current condition. Further, in order for self-blame to be adaptive (as had been reported in rape victims), it would need to be behavioral in nature. Such attributions would allow victims to feel a greater sense of control since future negative outcomes could be avoided by modifying behavior.

Janoff-Bulman (1979) presented empirical data in support of this hypothesis. She interviewed 48 rape counselors who reported that 74% of their clients blamed themselves in some way for their victimization experiences. Behavioral self-blame was reportedly much more common (69%) than characterological blame (19%), and in general, women who blamed their characters reported significantly greater levels of overall self-blame than those who reported behavioral self-blame. No indices of coping were obtained in this study and rape victims themselves were never questioned directly. Nevertheless, the attributions characteristic of rape victims were in direct contrast with those evident in a sample of depressed women assessed within the context of a second experiment reported by Janoff-Bulman (1979). Specifically, characterological self-blame characterized the depressed subjects and discriminated them from nondepressed women. As noted above, however, characterological blame was not very prevalent in rape victims, according to their counselors. These differential paterns of attribution were interpreted by Janoff-Bulman as supporting the necessity of discriminating between behavioral and characterological self-blame. Utilizing a single concept of self-blame in this study would have muddied the water by failing to differentiate possible adaptive and maladaptive roles of self-blame.

A subsequent analogue study provided support for the adaptive role of behavioral self-blame in rape victims (Janoff-Bulman, 1982). College females were asked to assume the role of either a rape victim or an observer of a sexual assault. They then listened to vignettes depicting such an assault and were asked to rate the degree of behavioral and/or characterological self-blame associated with the incident. These attributional ratings then were correlated with the degree to which subjects perceived the world to be under the influence of internal or external control (Rotter's Locus of Control Scale) and self-reported feelings of self-esteem.

Despite the weaknesses inherent in such an analogue design, results of Janoff-Bulman (1982) indicated that when subjects took the role of a rape victim, self-esteem was correlated positively and significantly only with behavioral blame. Alternatively, when the subjects rated blame from an observer's perspective, both types of self-blame were associated positively with higher esteem. These results suggested that only behavioral self-blame was adaptive for victims whereas both types of blame were adaptive for observers who allegedly could maintain perceptions of control over their own future outcomes by blaming the rape either on the actor's behavior or on her character. Behavioral self-blame was not associated directly with locus-of-control ratings, although the relationship between attribution and control was evident in the correlations between behavioral self-blame and perceived future avoidability. In particular, in both the victim and observer conditions, increased behavioral self-blame was associated with the belief that a similar situation could be avoided in the future. This relationship lends some credence to the notion that perceptions of control mediate attribution–coping relationships, though again, correlational analyses cannot lead definitively to such conclusions.

In a more recent study, a slightly different pattern of relationships emerged. In this study, Meyer and Taylor (1986) assessed 58 rape victims via anonymous questionnaires and found that most subjects reported some degree of self-blame. Only 37%, however, reported that self-blame was the primary cause for the incident, with 20% reporting characterological self-blame (e.g., they felt they had been too trusting) and 17% blaming their behavior (e.g., they believed they had been too careless). When attribution measures were factor analyzed, two self-blame factors emerged as exerting significant impacts on coping. These factors, "poor judgment" and "victim type," were described by the authors as being characteristic of behavioral and characterological blame respectively. The former included items evaluating blame relevant to the subject's behaviors and attitudes (e.g., "I made a rash decision," "I should have been more cautious") whereas the latter included items assessing unmodifiable personality characteristics (e.g., "I can't take care of myself" "I am a victim type").

Results indicated that both of these factors were correlated negatively with coping as measured by self-reported depressive symptoms, general ratings of fear, and satisfaction with sexual relationships (i.e., the higher the self-blame of any type, the poorer the coping). However, the "poor judgment" factor, described as an estimation of behavioral self-blame, included items defined a priori as being related to character. For example, "I am too trusting," which usually is characterized as a personality trait, loaded highly on the poor-judgment factor, apparently due to the fact that subjects perceived this personal characteristic as modifiable. "I am too impulsive" also loaded on the poor-judgment factor, although impulsivity traditionally has been viewed as a character trait. These data suggested that distinctions between behavioral and characterological blame are not as clear as they might appear.

Incest Victims

A second group of women who have experienced sexual trauma are incest victims. Silver et al. (1983) examined patterns of attribution and coping in a sample of these women and found that 20 years after their victimization experiences, 80% of the women were still searching for some meaning to attach to the event. The data also suggested that more active searches for meaning at the time of assessment were associated with poorer coping, although Silver et al. (1983) reported that no specific answers to a "Why me?" question were associated with measures of coping. It appeared that lack of meaning attached to the event was more debilitating than any particular type of attribution or interpretation of the event.[2] Specific attributional patterns were not assessed by Silver et al. (1983), however, and again results were correlational, thereby precluding any conclusions regarding causal relationships. Nevertheless, these data attested further to the importance of examining relationships between cognitive evaluations of victimization experiences and estimates of coping with such experiences.

Spouse-Abuse Victims

In a theoretical paper, Miller and Porter (1983) reviewed conceptual issues regarding the applicability of results reviewed above to victims of spouse abuse. Although victims of rape, incest, and spouse abuse can be perceived as having experienced similar traumatic events, Miller and Porter pointed out a number of unique aspects of the spouse-abuse situation that might lead to differential predictions regarding the influence of self-blame on coping in these individuals. First, victims of spouse abuse experience repeated assault from someone they know intimately. Second, they may not question, "Why me?" (vs. "Why not other people?") but, rather ask, "Why me *now*?" Third, self-blame in these women may take the form of evaluating ability to change a situation (e.g., "Why do I stay?" or "Why can't I change his behavior?") rather than estimating the degree to which one believes she was the cause of the earliest abuse (e.g., "What did I do to cause this?"). The nature of the questions asked could influence attributional perspectives in important ways. Finally, the repetitive nature of spouse abuse also may blur the distinction between behavioral and characterological blame. For example, if I perform the same behavior repeatedly, does that imply some evaluation of my personality? As will be discussed below, issues such as these are important in evaluating attribution–coping relationships and therefore should be the topic of future work in this area.

Chronic or Terminal Illness

A final area of victimization literature to be reviewed here involves victims of chronic or terminal illness. It is known that chronic disease can cause significant psychological maladjustment, and the role that attributions play in moderating such adjustment has been examined in samples of cancer and arthritis patients, as well as in mothers of children with diabetes and infants at high risk for developmental disability.

---

[2]Tait and Silver (in press) discussed more generally the importance of the search for meaning in effective coping with a variety of negative life events. Although review of their empirical findings and theoretical perspectives is beyond the scope of this chapter, the interested reader is referred to Tait and Silver for more extensive coverage of this topic.

Cancer Patients

Taylor, Lichtman, and Wood (1984) examined the roles of both self-blame and perceptions of control in a sample of 87 women with breast cancer. All but 3 of these patients had been treated surgically for their cancers between 1 and 60 months prior to the study. Patients were interviewed extensively and asked to complete various questionnaires in order to gather data regarding attributions about cancer onset, perceptions of control over the future course of the disorder, mood, self-esteem, and marital adjustment. Again, attributional responses differed depending on question format (open vs. closed), but 95% of the women reported having developed hypotheses about the causes of their cancers (open-ended format) and approximately 40% reported accepting some personal responsibility for onset of the cancers (closed-ended format). However, neither the presence of attributions about cancer onset (vs. absence of attributions) nor the presence of any particular attribution was related to enhanced levels of adjustment. (The only significant relationship reported was between blaming another person for cancer onset and poor adjustment. This pattern fits with Janoff-Bulman and Wortman's, 1977, just-world interpretation reviewed earlier, although correlational data could not rule out the alternative interpretation that maladjustment led to blaming someone else.) Most of the women also reported that deciding what had caused their cancers originally was not important, although the significance of assigning causality seemed to increase as time since surgery passed.

Despite the lack of significant relationships between attributions and coping with cancer, an important predictor of adjustment was perceived control. Perceptions that either oneself or another person (the physician) was in control of the subsequent course of the illness were significantly correlated with better adjustment. These data suggested that if an attribution–coping relationship exists in this population, perceived primary control over subsequent outcomes probably serves as a mediating variable. Such an hypothesis certainly is consistent with Kelley's early statements (see chap. 1) and with data discussed throughout this chapter.

Data from a study by Timko and Janoff-Bulman (1985) lent further empirical support to this control explanation. Namely, in a sample of 42 women also treated for breast cancer, attributions regarding the causes of cancer were not directly related to coping. However, attributions were related indirectly to adjustment in that attributions predicted perceived future avoidability and invulnerability (how likely am I to experience recurrence of this illness?), which in turn were significantly predictive of adjustment (as measured primarily by the Beck Depression Inventory).

Arthritis Patients

A complimentary pattern of results was reported with a sample of 55 male patients suffering from rheumatoid arthritis (Lowery, Jacobson, & Murphy, 1983). Namely, as in Taylor et al. (1984), the majority of patients (85%) reported that they had asked themselves the question, "Why me?," and had come up with a solution. Attributions reported via this open-ended procedure were coded according to their location along dimensions of locus, stability, and controllability. The most frequently given causes were classified as external, stable, and uncontrollable, although also as in Taylor et al. (1984), no significant relationship between attributions and adjustment occurred. Perceptions of control over the future course of the disorder were not assessed in this study, although it is possible that attributions influenced coping/adjustment only indirectly through effects on perceived control over similar future disabilities. It is unfortunate that such assessments were not conducted, but the control hypothesis certainly warrants further investigation in arthritic patients.

Parents of Chronically Ill or At-Risk Children

The relationship between attributions for physical illness and coping with disease also have been examined in parents of chronically ill or at-risk children. In these studies, the percentage of parents (typically mothers) who report having sought causal explanations for their childrens' physical difficulties range from 55% (Affleck, Tennen, & Gershman; 1985) to 85% (Affleck, Allen, Tennen, McGrade, & Ratzan, 1985). Across studies, approximately one-third of the mothers reported some degree of behavioral self-blame for their children's conditions (29.4%—Affleck, Allen, Tennen, McGrade, & Ratzan, 1985; 38.1%—Tennen, Affleck, & Gershman, 1986; and 30.2%—Affleck, Allen, McGrade, & McQueeney, 1982) and in two of these studies, behavioral self-blame was correlated positively with perceived or objective severity of the child's illness (Affleck, Allen, Tennen, McGrade, & Ratzan, 1985; Tennen, Affleck, & Gershman, 1986). However, relationships between behavioral self-blame and psychological adjustment in the mothers varied across studies.

In the study by Tennen et al. (1986), 50 mothers of infants with severe perinatal complications and who were judged to be at high risk for developmental disorders were interviewed in their homes shortly after hospital discharge. They were asked in an open-ended format what causes they felt might have been responsible for their children's difficulties and whether they felt that anything they had done might have been responsible for the severe medical problems. Mothers also estimated the degree of control they felt they would have over their infants' recoveries as well as the probability that similar problems would ensue with future pregnancies. Mother's mood was assessed as the primary measure of adjustment.

Results of correlational analyses in Tennen et al. (1986) were quite consistent with the Timko and Janoff-Bulman (1985) hypothesis described above. Behavioral self-blame was associated with perceived severity of the medical problems and also predicted subjects' estimates of their control over recurrence of the problem in subsequent pregnancies. Estimates of control over recurrence in turn predicted level of mood. In other words, mothers who were better adapted emotionally felt behaviorally responsible for their infants' problems and were more likely to feel in control over the possibility that similar difficulties would result from future pregnancies. This pattern of results again suggested that the effects of attributional activity on coping with disease were moderated by their impact on perceived avoidability or control over future outcomes. However, Tennen et al. presented at least one plausible alternative hypothesis for these data. Specifically, as mothers perceived their children's physical problems to be more severe, they may have become more distressed and therefore more likely to search extensively for causal explanations. A more extensive search could lead to increased likelihood of behavioral blame, hence the relationship between severity and self-blame. Alternate explanations such as this certainly merit further attention given the correlational nature of the data currently available.

A second study with a similar population of mothers failed to demonstrate a positive relationship between self-blame and coping with infants' severe perinatal complications (Affleck et al., 1982). Nevertheless, this study reported a complimentary negative relationship between blaming others and emotional adjustment. Namely, blaming other people for the infants' problems (e.g., obstetric error, insufficient stimulation in the intensive care unit) was associated with increased mood disturbance and enhanced anticipation of difficulties expected to occur with caregiving for the infant in the future. Affleck et al. (1982) did not address the relationship between attributional activity and perceived control, however.

In a third study with mothers of infants at risk for developmental disabilities, Affleck, Tennen, and Gershman (1985) found a positive relationship between the presence of attributions regarding the medical problems (vs. absence of such) and mood. In other words, mothers who had settled on some cause for their infants' difficulties were more emotionally well-adjusted than mothers who had found no answer to the "Why me?" question. In this same study, mothers also were better adjusted emotionally if they perceived some control over future recurrence of the problem. However, the relationship between attributions and perceived future control was not reported, and none of these mothers reported any explanations that involved self-blame. Rather, they attributed their infants' problems to fate, bad luck, or some alternative purpose. Hence, the relationship between self-blame, control, and coping in mothers of at-risk infants requires further examination.

These relationships also were investigated in a sample of parents with children suffering from insulin-dependent diabetes (Affleck, Allen, Tennen, McGrade, & Ratzan, 1985). Mothers of diabetic children were asked about their attributions regarding onset of the disorder, whether they had ever asked and/or answered the question, "Why me?," and how severely they perceived the symptoms to be in their children. The treating endocrinologist and clinic-nurse educators associated with each family rated the mother's adjustment on a 5-point rating scale. Eighty-five percent of the mothers reported having asked the question, "Why me?," with answers falling into the following categories: God's will, punishment, and selection (e.g., "I guess I was selected to have this happen to my child; I'm the type that can handle something like this"). Two-thirds of the sample reported benefits from having a diabetic child, and attributions fell into four categories—heredity, environment, physiological causes, and behavioral self-blame—with heredity and environment the most frequently cited causes. Twenty-nine percent of the mothers reported some behavioral self-blame for their children's diabetic condition, and these ratings were significantly correlated with perceived severity of the disorder. However, the only relationship between attribution and adjustment involved a significant correlation between attribution of the illness to environmental factors and more optimal ratings of coping—that is, mothers were rated as being better adjusted if they attributed the diabetes to environmental factors (e.g., stressful circumstances). Perception of control over symptoms was not related to adjustment in this study.

These data require replication in order to clarify the utility of the control hypothesis with parents of diabetic children. A number of variables differ between this patient population and infants at risk for developmental disorders. For instance, age of the patient, the parents' level of past experience with parenting, and the nature of the negative outcomes expected all differ. These variables will need to be taken into account in any further attempts to apply results from other studies to this population.

Concluding Points

In the psychological literature, victims are defined as persons who have experienced some type of life change as a result of severe psychological or physical loss. Common reactions to victimization include anxiety, helplessness, loss of self-esteem, rumination, loss of meaning, and depression. It has been suggested that the experience of victimization leads to initiation of a search for causes of the event in order to restore beliefs in a just, orderly, and/or controllable world. Although restoration of these beliefs can occur in a number of ways, this section reviewed the ways in which attributions of the event facilitate or inhibit adjustment to victimization.

We reviewed data addressing the attribution–coping relationship in victims of physical injury, sexual assault, and chronic or terminal illness. These groups certainly are only subsets, however, of the many individuals who suffer severe losses and attempt to make sense of their plights through attributional activity. As reviewed in chapter 5, for example, people who experience loss of a close relationship (through death of a partner, separation, or divorce) often develop attributional stories or accounts to make sense of their experience (Weber et al., 1987; Weiss, 1975). Accounts of traumatic events also are made by groups such as Vietnam veterans and adolescent prostitutes (Harvey, Agostinelli, & Weber, 1988).

Limiting ourselves to the populations examined here, however, a positive relationship between attributing the victimizing event to one's past behavior (behavioral self-blame) and effective coping was reported in victims of severe physical injury and sexual assault. Attributing the event to others was associated at times with poorer coping. These relationships did not occur consistently, and opposite patterns were demonstrated. For example, in some groups behavioral self-blame was associated with poorer coping (Kiecolt-Glaser & Williams, 1987). Moreover, the percentages of victims who actually blamed themselves for their experiences varied across studies.

Despite inconsistent empirical patterns, one of the most plausible hypotheses given the data currently available is that relationships between attribution and coping in victims may be mediated by perceptions of the probability that the trauma could have been avoided and beliefs about the degree to which victims feel in control over similar future outcomes/events. However, this hypothesis is far from definitive and may not be appropriate for all types of victims.

Theoretical and Methodological Issues

Possible reasons for discrepancies in the literature have been reviewed in the text above, but these will be reiterated and elaborated upon here. Four categories of variables that may influence empirical relationships between attributions and coping in victims of various traumas will be explored: (a) methods of measuring attribution, (b) methods of assessing coping or adjustment, (c) nature of the victimization experience, and (d) personality variables.

Measurement of Attributions

Across the studies reviewed above, a number of methods were used to assess attributions in vitims. One major measurement difference concerned the use of open- versus closed-ended questions. As Turnquist et al. (1988) noted, closed-ended questions (e.g., rating scales) allow easier scoring of attributions but also limit subjects to causal choices proposed by the experimenter. Such a strategy may force an individual to choose a specific cause for an event when he/she actually would prefer to think of the cause as ambiguous (Snyder & Wicklund, 1981). Open-ended responses, on the other hand, allow subjects the freedom to generate causes although they typically require that some kind of coding scheme be imposed to make sense of the data. These coding schemes often are inconsistent across studies (Turnquist et al., 1988) and again may promote the appearance of attributional specificity when it does not necessarily exist.

One example of such difficulties occurred in Tennen et al. (1986). When parents of children at high risk for developmental disorders were asked in an open-ended format what causes they thought might be responsible for their children's difficulties, the most frequently cited attributions were coded as representing behavioral self-blame. When these same parents were asked to rate on 10-point scales the degree to which various causes were responsible, chance was rated higher than either the parents' own or others' behavior.

The format of open-ended questions also may influence empirical outcomes. In some reports, open-ended measures took the form of asking subjects to respond to the question, "Why me?" It was clear from subjects' responses that this form of question did not always elicit solely attributional material. In response to this question, subjects at times cited benefits of the trauma. Hence, attributional responses to this question might be expected to vary in nature and frequency from ratings provided for different open-ended formats (e.g., "Why did this happen?") as well as for specific attributional self-report items.

Of more theoretical interest is Shaver and Drown's (1986) critique of attributional measures. These authors provided a cogent argument that divergences in the victimization literature may result from an inappropriate interchangeability of the terms *cause*, *responsibility*, and *blame*. Numerous papers reviewed above were cited by Shaver and Drown (1986) as using these terms interchangeably. For example, Taylor et al. (1984) asked subjects to attribute responsibility for their cancer to various factors, but discussed their results in terms of blame. Also, Tennen et al. (1986) used both cause and responsibility interchangeably in the same question. As will be recalled from discussions in chapters 1 and 4, distinctions between these terms should not be ignored. To reiterate, causes can be described relative to positive *or* negative outcomes, and they are defined as any antecedents to an event or an effect that are sufficient for the event or effect to occur. Responsibility and blame, on the other hand, are typically associated only with negative outcomes. The assignment of responsibility depends on an individual's intent to cause the outcome, his/her awareness that such an outcome would occur, and appreciation of moral wrongdoing in bringing about the event. Attribution of blame is dependent upon one's perception that a causal individual is giving a poor "excuse" that his/her behavior was unintentional. Given investigators' confusion of these differential definitions, Shaver and Drown argued that no coherent picture of attribution in victimization can be drawn.

Measurement of Coping

The studies reviewed above varied with regard to the strategies used for assessing coping with victimization. In some studies, coping was defined as emotional adjustment and was assessed with various mood inventories (e.g., Lowery et al., 1983; Tennen et al., 1986; Timko & Janoff-Bulman,

1985). In other papers, coping was defined as compliance with a medical regimen (Kiecolt-Glaser & Williams, 1987), while in still others coping was rated in a global fashion (Janoff-Bulman & Wortman, 1977; Taylor et al., 1984). In addition, coping measures were sometimes rated by the subjects themselves and at other times by medical staff (Janoff-Bulman & Wortman, 1977) or interviewers (Taylor et al., 1984). As Wortman (1983) emphasized, different assessments of coping need not be correlated with each other.

As noted by Turnquist et al. (1988), the choice of an appropriate outcome measure should be based on knowledge of the base rates of various coping strategies that typically follow the illness/injury in question. If a particular outcome is quite prevalent for all individuals who suffer a traumatic event (e.g., smoking cessation that typically occurs following heart attack; Croog & Richards, 1977), relevant attributions (e.g., attribution of the heart attack to smoking) may have no additional power to predict coping responses. In general, a thorough conceptualization of coping probably should include evaluations of adjustment along a number of dimensions such as psychiatric symptomatology, emotional well-being, effective functioning in social, familial, and occupational spheres, physical health, and global quality of life (Wortman, 1983).

Nature of Victimization

Diseases, sexual assault, and accidents by nature may suggest differential attribution–coping links. This suggestion comes from the awareness that these events differ with regard to the degree to which others are necessarily involved and therefore can be implicated as causal agents. In particular, sexual assault requires participation from another person whereas accidents may occur when one is alone or with someone else. Diseases such as cancer are typically experienced alone. Traumatic events also differ with regard to the most plausible explanations associated with each—for example, accidents are by definition associated with some degree of chance. Not only the nature of the event, but also the severity of the outcome (e.g., pervasiveness of physical disability) may influence attribution–coping relationships (Kiecolt-Glaser & Williams, 1987). Miller and Porter (1983) suggested a similar influential variable when they discussed the repetitive nature of spouse abuse and its likely impact on attribution–coping relationships. Thus, attribution–victimization researchers cannot ignore differences inherent in the nature or severity of traumatic experiences and the possible influence of these on the effects and/or correlates of attributions.

Personality Variables

Attribution–coping links in victims may be mediated by personality variables. For example, certain personality types may be more likely to experience a particular type of trauma. As previously discussed, for example, spinal-cord-injury patients are more likely than burn patients to be young males with high degrees of risk-taking personality characteristics (Kiecolt-Glaser & Williams, 1987). Such traits may influence the types of attributions made in response to victimization or may moderate the impact of these on coping. In addition, individual differences in people who all experience the same type of trauma may have an impact on the nature and effects of attributions. For instance, individual differences in attributional style may influence interpretations of and responses to traumatic events (Peterson & Seligman, 1983). It has been noted that some people are more likely to accept responsibility for negative events in general. These people, therefore, would be expected to respond similarly to victimizing experiences. Thus, individual differences may account for some of the variability in coping since not all victims respond to their experiences in the same way. While some victims are likely to become passive in response to their experiences, others are more apt to become activists for a cause (Peterson & Seligman, 1983). (See chap. 9 for additional discussions regarding individual differences in attribution.)

Smoking Cessation

In other areas of health psychology, individuals who are the topic of study are less likely to be perceived as victims. Smokers are one such group. These people are not perceived as victims since they usually have not experienced significant life change due to some psychological or physical loss (although they often are perceived as being at risk for such losses). However, given the significant health hazards associated with smoking, a large body of work has addressed the effects of various treatment interventions for smoking cessation. Within this literature, a small number of studies have examined the relationship between attributions and smokers' ability to stop smoking or remain abstinent following smoking-cessation treatment.

Smoking cessation at times has been defined as an achievement behavior, with inability to quit smoking or remain abstinent considered a "failure" and cessation or abstinence characterized as a "success" (Weiner, 1986; see chap. 9 for additional information regarding achievement–attribution relationships). In this light, smoking cessation differs extensively from victimization in that positive or negative outcomes can be associated with the former whereas the latter implies a loss, or negative outcome.

Attribution and Treatment Outcome

In at least one study (Harackiewicz, Sansone, Blair, Epstein, & Manderlink, 1987), smokers demonstrated a self-serving bias (see chap. 2 & 9) following treatment. At the end of treatment, ex-smokers (who had "succeeded" in stopping smoking) attributed their treatment outcomes more to internal causes (ability to quit, the challenge of quitting, personal effort) than smokers (who had "failed" to stop). In addition, smokers attributed their treatment outcomes more frequently to external causes (their doctor, an unexpected event) than ex-smokers. In other words, success was attributed more to internal causes whereas failure was attributed to external variables.

Harackiewicz et al. (1987) also reported that attributions varied somewhat as a function of the mode of treatment. In their study, subjects underwent smoking-cessation treatment with or without the assistance of nicotine gum, the use of which should be expected to convey external cause. All subjects also were given a "self-help manual" to aid their progress through treatment. Instructions within this manual varied such that either internal or external perspectives on treatment were emphasized. For example, "internal instructions" emphasized statements such as, "Your determination and effort will be most important in becoming a nonsmoker" (Harackiewicz et al., 1987, p. 374). "External instructions" included statements such as, "Following the guidelines of this program will be most important in becoming a nonsmoker" (p. 374).

These instructions were expected to influence attributions for treatment outcome, but these expectations were only partially confirmed. External attributions for smokers (failure) and internal attributions for ex-smokers (success) were equally high regardless of treatment condition. In other words, attributions consistent with a self-serving bias were apparently unaffected by treatment instructions. On the other hand, instructions to make internal attributions had an effect on attributions in smokers (failure) whereas external instructions had an impact on attributions of ex-smokers (success)—that is, when attributions were not consistent with the self-serving pattern, instructions regarding the most likely causes for improvement had an impact on subjects' attributions regardless of the actual treatment mode (presence or absence of nicotine gum).

Further data from the same study (Harackiewicz et al., 1987) indicated that treatment gains were maximized when there was a match between the attributions made by subjects and the primary mode of treatment. In other words, when subjects were given nicotine gum (an external factor) to aid in their cessation treatment, maintenance of abstinence was greater if these individuals made external rather than internal attributions for their outcomes. Subjects who made external attributions when treatment did not entail use of an explicit external intervention did not fare as well as those who made internal attributions under those conditions.

Attributions and Relapse

In addition to gathering information regarding the typical patterns of attributions that occur in smokers and ex-smokers following treatment, it is important to consider the impact that these cognitions have on subsequent relapse or continued abstinence during a follow-up period. Goldstein, Gordon, and Marlatt (1984) reported that following treatment, smokers were more likely to relapse if they attributed an initial incident of smoking (a "slip" during the follow-up phase) to internal, stable, and global causes. These data are consistent with work reviewed in chapter 9 suggesting that stable and global attributions are associated with lower expectancies for future success, which in turn should lead to a greater chance of future relapse (Weiner, 1986). In addition, internal attributions for an initial "slip" could result in reduced self-esteem for the smoker who has been unable to remain abstinent, and this lowered esteem also could make it more difficult to remain abstinent (Weiner, 1986).

More recent data were supportive of the link between attributions, expectations, and continued abstinence from smoking. In one large-scale study, for example, Eiser and colleagues (Eiser & van der Pligt, 1986; Eiser, van der Pligt, Raw, & Sutton, 1985) mailed questionnaires to over 2,000 smokers. Information about their attributions for other smokers' failure to quit, subjects' own intentions to try to quit, and confidence in (expectancies about) their own abilities to stop smoking were elicited. One year later, approximately 1,800 of the individuals were recontacted, again through mailed questionnaires, and queried regarding any attempts to quit during the intervening 12 months and about their current smoking status (smoking or abstinent). Path analyses then were conducted to examine the relationships between cognitions at time 1 (i.e., attributions, expectations or confidence, and intentions) and behavior at time 2 (i.e., smoking behavior during and at the end of the subsequent 12 months).

Results of both studies indicated that internal attributions for others' failure to quit were unrelated to any of the other variables. However, attributing others' failure to quit to stable factors was related inversely to subjects' confidence in their own abilities to quit. If subjects thought that others were unable to quit for reasons that were unmodifiable or stable (e.g., difficulty of the task, person type) they were less confident that they themselves would be able to stop smoking. Ratings of self-confidence then were significantly predictive of intentions to quit—that is, lower confidence was associated with less intention to quit. Further, intentions to quit predicted both actual attempts to quit during the 12 months (tried vs. did not try) and smoking status at the end of the follow-up period (smoking or abstinent). These data suggested that although attributions did not relate directly to smoking behavior, they may have influenced smoking status indirectly through their impact on expectations and intentions.

The pattern of data from the studies by Eiser and colleagues is consistent with research on smoking in self-efficacy theory (Bandura, 1977, 1982). Self-efficacy expectancies, or confidence in one's abilities to refrain from smoking, are significantly predictive of smoking relapse during various follow-up periods (Condiotte & Lichtenstein, 1981; DiClemente, Prochaska, & Gibertini, 1985). As will be discussed in chapter 9, however, these studies do not address directly the attributional components that make up self-efficacy expectancies.

Concluding Points

The data available, although limited, suggest that attributions may have a significant impact on smoking behavior. Future work should include replications of these studies as well as additional projects to address unanswered questions regarding the interactions between other factors (e.g., personality variables, general health attitudes, physical-health status) and attributions on smoking behavior.

Type A Personality Style

An additional area of interest to attribution–health researchers that also does not fall under the rubric of victimization concerns the relationship between the Type A behavior pattern and coronary disease. The Type A behavior pattern was first described by Friedman and Rosenman (1974) and since that time has received extensive empirical and popular attention. Type A individuals have been described as exhibiting a consistent pattern of hard-driving, competitive behavior. They also have been characterized as impatient, time-urgent, and easily angered when situations or other people hinder their attempts to achieve. Although specific risk ratios vary (Matthews & Haynes, 1986) it generally appears that Type A individuals are twice as likely to develop coronary disease as Type B persons, defined as those without the characteristics of a Type A pattern (e.g., Review Panel, 1981).

Although Type A individuals are at higher risk for experiencing physical trauma than Type Bs (as are smokers compared to nonsmokers), they typically are not considered to be victims. Thus, study of the Type A pattern has not come from a victimization perspective. Rather, of interest in the majority of Type A work are the mechanisms through which this behavioral pattern leads to increased incidence of coronary disease. In a subset of this work, a number of papers have investigated the role of attributions in the demonstration and maintenance of this behavioral pattern. It is this sub-body of work that will be addressed here.

Type A Personality and Desire for Control

One of the primary theoretical perspectives regarding the Type A personality style involves the notion that Type A behavior represents a means of coping with uncontrollable stimuli (Glass, 1977).[3] Within this perspective, Type As are perceived as being more concerned than Type Bs with maintaining control. Empirical data have supported this perspective showing that compared to Type Bs, Type As have a greater desire for control, are more reluctant to give up control to others, and demonstrate different behavioral patterns when they are faced with a loss of control (see Strube, 1987, for a review of these studies). All empirical work has not been supportive of the control perspective, however, and attributional data that might corroborate the theory have been mixed.

If the behavior of Type As were motivated by a desire for control, patterns of attributions should demonstrate what has been called a control bias, with Type As attributing their behavior more often then Type Bs to factors under their control. Some data have supported such a conception. For example, Brunson and Matthews (1981) asked college subjects to perform a concept-formation task with which they experienced uncontrollable failure. Upon completion of the task, subjects rated the degree to which various causes were responsible for their performance. In response to these questions, Type As attributed their failure more to internal causes (e.g., ability, effort) over which they apparently perceived control, while Type Bs attributed their failure more to external causes over which they had no control (e.g., task difficulty, chance, and the experimenter). Thus, it appeared that As exhibited a control bias whereas Bs demonstrated a self-serving bias.

Despite the apparent support that these data provided for the control hypothesis, other data from the same study were not corroborative. Prior to making the above ratings, subjects had been asked to verbalize their thoughts during task performance. Results suggested that when lack of control was salient (subjects were asked to write down the results of all trials on which they failed and thus were acutely aware of their repeated experience with failure), Type As attributed failure more frequently to lack of ability than Type Bs. On the other hand, when lack of control was less salient (subjects only heard orally the results of their trials), attributions to ability were equal for Type As and Bs. These data suggested that the relationship between attribution, control, and Type A style is not a simple one and may depend on situational variables.

Other data supporting the control hypothesis were reported by Rhodewalt (1984). In this study, 40 health-care professionals completed the Attributional Style Questionnaire (ASQ) (Seligman, Abramson, Sem-

---

[3] Strube (1988) reviewed other major theoretical interpretations of the Type A behavior pattern. However, these will not be discussed here since the control perspective has been the primary source of attributional theories within this literature. Interested readers are advised to read Strube (1988) for an introduction to other major hypotheses.

mel, & Von Baeyer, 1979; see chap. 7 for a fuller discussion of this instrument). Subjects characterized as Type A attributed both positive and negative outcomes to internal and stable causes whereas Type Bs attributed only positive outcomes in such a way. The latter group, on the other hand, attributed negative outcomes to external, unstable causes. These data again seemed to demonstrate that Type A individuals were biased to attribute causes such that all outcomes, whether positive or negative, were experienced as being under personal control (control bias). On the other hand, Type Bs exhibited a self-serving bias, attributing only positive outcomes to personal variables.

Other data have implied a somewhat different story. A study by Strube (1985) utilized a methodology similar to that reported by Rhodewalt (1984) in which college subjects characterized as Type A or B responded to hypothetical situations via the ASQ. In this study, a composite attribution score was calculated for each subject by averaging subjects' ratings of causes along internal, stable, and global dimensions. Results indicated that Type As responded with a self-serving rather than a control bias. Both Type As and Bs took more credit for positive than for negative outcomes, but the effect was more pronounced in Type As. The results were not completely conclusive, however, since in one of the experiments reported by Strube (1985), this self-serving bias occurred only for male Type As.

In a separate study (Strube & Boland, 1986), college subjects were given success or failure experiences with anagram tasks. Again, a self-serving bias was exhibited by individuals characterized as Type A. Strube and Boland (1986) reported that Type As made more internal attributions for success than for failure whereas Type Bs made more external attributions for success than failure. It is unclear from the presentation of results, however, what significance levels were attained with these comparisons.

Explanations for Empirical Inconsistencies

As a result of these inconsistencies in the data, it is unclear whether or not a desire for control serves a central role in the attributional patterns for Type A individuals. It may be that desire for control is manifested at times by a self-serving pattern of attributions, while at other times by consistently internal attributions (what has been called the control bias). Situational variables may determine, for example, whether one feels more in control by attributing failure to oneself or to external variables. Depending on the situation, either of these patterns could imply that an individual will be able to revise some aspect of self or the environment in order to exert control in subsequent experiences with the same task.

Strube (1987) proposed a theoretical interpretation of the Type A behavior pattern that might explain the lack of consistency in attributional patterns. He suggested that the primary motivating force behind the Type A pattern is a need to maintain certainty about one's ability level. Further, lack of control may be only one of a number of situations that lead Type As to question their abilities, and therefore only one of a variety of situations that might elicit Type A behavior. Strube (1987) reviewed a significant amount of data in support of this hypothesis and suggested that the self-serving attributional pattern exhibited by Type As in his work (e.g., Strube, 1985; Strube & Boland, 1986) supports his "self-appraisal model." Namely, a self-serving pattern should enhance beliefs in one's abilities since successes are attributed to ability but failure is not attributed to the lack thereof.

Although it is not entirely clear that the self-serving pattern is as consistent as Strube suggests, his ideas regarding the impact of such an attributional style fit with clinical impressions of the relationship between Type A behavior and health. For example, Strube (1987, 1988) reported that a self-serving pattern may hinder Type As from realizing that they lack ability in some area or may contribute to an inability to generalize their limitations to new situations. Hence, in their constant striving for positive self-appraisal they may continue attempts to achieve under conditions in which such striving is inappropriate. As a result, they create unnecessary stress for themselves.

Methodological differences in the assessment of attribution also have been posited to explain empirical inconsistencies. Strube (1988) suggested that evaluation of causal sources (e.g., ability, effort—as in Brunson and Matthews, 1981) may lead to very different results from assessments of causal dimensions (as in Strube, 1985) given that Type As may vary in their interpretations of causes along these dimensions. Strube (1988) provided some data in support of his hypothesis. College subjects were given either success or failure experiences with anagram tasks and rated the degree to which effort and ability were responsible for their performances. They also were asked to rate these causes along internality, stability, and generality dimensions. Results indicated that Type A students attributed failure more to effort than Type B students, appearing to indicate a self-blaming, control bias. However, under these conditions, Type As also perceived effort to be a less stable cause than Type Bs, suggesting a pattern of results that more closely approximates a self-serving pattern (e.g., "I failed, but not due to anything that is going to make me fail again.")

Strube's data (1988) did not fully explain inconsistencies in the literature. First, his conclusions were limited given that he failed to ask subjects to rate the influence of external causes. Second, in the study by Rhodewalt (1984), subjects also were asked to make dimensional ratings of attributions and support for a self-blaming, control bias was demonstrated with these measures. Hence, other explanations are warranted. Additional methodological differences across studies, for example, have included differential quantitative cutoffs for identifying Type A and B individuals, different methods of defining success and failure (hypothetical vs. laboratory analogue procedures), and minor differences in age and gender distributions of subjects.

Individual Differences

Individual differences in attributional style or desire for control among Type As may moderate the relationship between Type A behavior and coronary illness. As Strube (1987) noted, not all Type A individuals are coronary-prone, and it may be that only Type As with certain attributional patterns (e.g., a self-serving bias, a control bias) are more likely to experience coronary problems.

Data exist in support of the individual-difference conception, although the degree to which these support the self-appraisal model or the control hypothesis is unclear. In two studies by Rhodewalt and colleagues, apparent noncompliance with medical regimens among Type As was related to increased self-attribution for the medical problems. Type As with running-related injuries (Rhodewalt & Strube, 1985) and others with insulin-dependent diabetes (Rhodewalt & Marcroft, 1988) were assessed. In both studies, Type As who appeared to be noncompliant with treatment (e.g., runners whose doctors viewed them as progressing less well through treatment and diabetics whose blood glucose levels displayed inadequate control over diabetes) reported feeling more responsible for their medical conditions than Type As who appeared to be compliant with treatment. The noncompliant patients also reported more desire to "fight the injury," more anger over their conditions, and somewhat less desire to participate in a medical regimen.

These data were interpreted by the authors as supporting hypotheses from a control perspective since at least a subset of Type As seemed to respond to medical treatment with reactance. In other words, these Type As perceived that compliance with a medical regimen would require them to relinquish control. In reactance to this perception, they assumed control over the medical problem themselves (by self-attributing), indicated the need to fight the problem on their own (perhaps also to regain control), and expressed anger toward the problem that threatened their sense of control.

The data were not completely consistent with this interpretation, however. First, self-attributions in Rhodewalt and Strube (1985) were made in a global manner without attention to their dimensional structure. Second, Rhodewalt and Marcroft (1988) reported that noncompliant Type As did not differ from compliant As or Bs in general attributional style—that is, they did attribute not positive or negative outcomes differently with regard to internality, stability, or globality. Also in this latter study, noncompliant Type As did not report enchanced desire for control compared to the other two groups.

Concluding Points

In general, these data suggest that attributional activity may have an important role to play in the relationship between Type A behavior and health-related functioning. However, the nature and meaning of this relationship is still somewhat unclear. Specifically, the nature of attributional activity in Type As seems inconsistent, and the degree to which desire for control (or some other motivation such as self-appraisal) activates the Type A pattern and influences attributions is unknown. Also, the role of individual differences in attributional style or motivation for control is uncertain. Hence, this area is a fertile arena for future attributional work.

General Concluding Points

The victimization literature, although not entirely consistent, suggests that attributions often are significantly related to coping with traumatic events such as physical injury, sexual assault, or chronic illness. General conclusions indicate that it probably is better to have found some explanation for the event than to be in a state of uncertainty (although it was noted that under some circumstances attributional ambiguity may be associated with more adequate adjustment). Also, explanations that provide individuals with a sense of control over future outcomes probably lead to (or at least are associated with) improved coping. However, additional research certainly is required to specify the impact on coping of variables such as the precise nature of the trauma and personality characteristics of the individual traumatized on various modes of coping.

When individuals are less likely to be perceived as victims (as in smokers and Type A individuals), relationships between attributions and behavior also are important. Specifically, attributions for smoking cessation are associated with treatment outcome and relapse, and attributional patterns in Type A individuals may moderate the relationship between this behavioral pattern and coronary disease or may have an impact on compliance with medical regimens.

The relationships between attributions and health-related functioning reviewed in this chapter attest to the importance of continued study in the attribution–health domain. The significant relationships described suggest that attributional activity could be a useful target for psychological intervention following various modes of traumatization and during treatment for health-related behavior such as smoking. Attributions also could be a target of programs designed to reduce the likelihood of heart disease in persons characterized as Type A. Prior to the implementation of such treatment programs, however, more will need to be learned regarding the causal relationship between attributions and health-related behavior. If indeed attributions have a causal impact on health behavior, intervention at the attributional level could prove quite vital to health promotion and maintenance as well as coping with health-related problems.

7
Attributional Processes and the Development of Dysfunctional Behaviors

Within the last 20 years there has been an increasing tendency for theorists and researchers to acknowledge the importance of social–cognitive processes in the acquisition and maintenance of dysfunctional behaviors (e.g., Arnkoff & Mahoney, 1979; Bandura, 1977; Leary & Miller, 1986; Meichenbaum, 1977; Weary & Mirels, 1982; Wortman & Brehm, 1975). Of particular interest has been the notion that cognitions about oneself may serve as mediators in the maintenance and modification of various behavior patterns. For example, response–outcome expectations (Seligman, 1975), efficacy expectations (Bandura, 1977), self-instructions (Meichenbaum, 1977), and self-statements (Ellis, 1962) have all been proposed as mechanisms involved in the pathogenesis, maintenance, and therapeutic treatment of a variety of behavioral disorders. Many of these cognitive explanations of dysfunctional behaviors involve attributional activities, and in this chapter we will examine empirical evidence relevant to the possible role of attributional processes in the development of clinically relevant target behaviors. In particular, we will examine attributional activities as they relate to Seligman's (e.g., Abramson et al., 1978) learned-helplessness model of depression and to Storms and McCaul's (1976) model of the emotional exacerbation of dysfunctional behaviors. We will end our discussion with a treatment of research examining the notion that psychological symptoms may be used strategically to protect esteem.

An Attributional Analysis of Learned Helplessness and Depression

Depression is a disorder of the entire psychobiological system (Burns & Beck, 1978) and generally involves somatic, emotional, and behavioral disturbances. Somatic symptoms of depression, for example, may include loss of sleep, appetite, or sexual desire. In addition, feelings of sadness, guilt, and despair, behavioral passivity, inactivity, and social withdrawal are characteristic of depressive disorders. The following account was given by a clinically-depressed female and illustrates many of the disturbances commonly reported by depressed individuals.

> I can sum up my problems very easily. I'm a total failure in life. Nothing I do seems to work out. My married life is dull. My husband and I rarely do things together anymore—except argue. He just seems to be disinterested in me, and probably with good reason. Neither of my children are doing well in school. I know I should try to help them and try to be more supportive, but I just don't. I get mad and yell at them. I just don't have what it takes to be a good mother—or wife, I guess. Even my work is drudgery; my successes at work seem meaningless to me. I'm so tired. I don't have the energy to do much of anything. I really feel that my life is hopeless. I'd be better off dead. My family would be better off too if I were out of the picture.

It is clear from this account that the woman feels helpless and views most of her negative life outcomes as due to something about her. Her life, as she describes it, is a series of failures for which she is responsible.

Seligman and his associates have proposed that feelings of helplessness and attributions of self-blame interfere with the ability to respond adaptively to stressful situations and are important in the development of depression in humans. Before discussing Seligman's model of depression, however, we should point out that the model of learned helplessness was originally formulated on the basis of laboratory studies with dogs and other nonhuman animals. For this reason, it is necessary to discuss the basic experimental paradigm used in learned-helplessness research with animals.

In most of Seligman's early studies of the learned-helplessness phenomenon (Overmier & Seligman, 1967; Seligman & Maier, 1967; Seligman, Maier, & Geer, 1968), animals were exposed, during a "pretreatment" phase, to controllable shocks, uncontrollable shocks, or no pretreatment. They subsequently were placed in a shuttlebox containing two compartments separated by a barrier. In each experimental trial, a signal was presented for 10 seconds prior to the administration of an electrical shock. If the animal jumped the barrier during the signal period or after the shock began, the receipt of electrical shock could be avoided altogether or escaped. On the next experimental trial, the animal was required to jump back across the barrier in order to avoid or escape the signalled shock. In general, the results of studies using this general paradigm have indicated that relative to animals in the controllable-shock or pretreatment-control conditions, animals who were pretreated with uncontrollable, inescapable shock failed during experimental trials to avoid or escape from the electrical shocks. Instead, these animals tolerated extreme amounts of shock passively.

This interference with escape–avoidance behaviors produced in animals by prior inescapable shock has been termed "learned helplessness." Seligman (1973, 1975) has contended that the major causal factor in the development of learned helplessness is the organism's belief or expectancy that its responses will not influence the future probability of environmental outcomes (expectancy of response–outcome independence). According to Seligman, Maier, and Solomon (1971):

S makes active responses during exposure to inescapable shocks. Because shock cannot be controlled, S learns that shock termination is independent of its behavior. S's incentive for initiating active instrumental responses during a shock is assumed to be partially produced by its having learned that the probability of shock termination will be increased by these responses. When this expectation is absent, the incentive for instrumental responding should be reduced. The presence of shock in the escape-avoidance training situation should then arouse the same expectation that was previously acquired during exposure to inescapable shocks: shock is uncontrollable. Therefore, the incentive for initiating and maintaining active instrumental responses in the training situation should be low. . . . In addition, learning that shock termination and responding are independent should interfere with the subsequent association of responding and shock termination. . . . More exposures to the new contingency should be required in order for S to learn that shock is controllable, because S has already learned that shock is uncontrollable. This is why we think preshocked dogs have difficulty acquiring escape and avoidance responding even after they once jump the barrier and terminate the shock (p. 369).

While a number of alternative explanations have been offered as explanations for the learning deficits that result from exposure to uncontrollable outcomes (see Maier & Seligman, 1976, for a review), the learned-helplessness interpretation has received the most attention and has been the most widely investigated.

Following the early helplessness experiments with animals, a number of researchers investigated the occurrence, nature, and parameters of learned helplessness in humans (Hiroto, 1974; Hiroto & Seligman, 1975; Klein, Fencil-Morse, & Seligman, 1976; Roth & Bootzin, 1974). Many of these studies of human helplessness attempted to reproduce the animal findings in humans (Abramson et al., 1978). For example, Hiroto (1974) assigned college students to a controllable-noise, an uncontrollable-noise, or a no-noise training condition. In the test phase of the experiment, all subjects were tested for helplessness in an apparatus analogous to the shuttlebox used in animal research. In the shuttlebox, all subjects were informed that a loud noise would come on periodically but that they could terminate the noise by moving a lever from one side of the shuttlebox to the other. Consistent with the results of animal-helplessness experiments, Hiroto (1974) found that subjects who had previously been exposed to uncontrollable noise failed to escape the noise during the test phase, while controllable- and no-noise subjects readily learned the escape–avoidance response.

Similar performance deficits for subjects exposed to uncontrollable outcomes in the test phase of experiments concerned with human helplessness have been found by other investigators; it is important to note, however, that several studies have found increases in performance following learned-helplessness training (e.g., Roth & Bootzin, 1974; Roth & Kubal, 1975). In an attempt to explain such "facilitation effects," Wortman and Brehm (1975) have suggested that when individuals who expect to have control over their outcomes are exposed to uncontrollable outcomes, they will experience psychological reactance (Brehm, 1966, 1972) and will exhibit increased motivation to exert control and improved performance. But through repeated exposure to uncontrollable outcomes, they will learn they cannot control their outcomes and will exhibit the performance deficits characteristic of learned helplessness.

A somewhat different explanation for the performance-enhancement versus -decrement findings has been advanced by Pittman and D'Agostino (1985). Specifically, they proposed that following exposure to uncontrollable outcomes, individuals are motivated to protect against further loss of control and self-esteem and that this motivation induces a careful and precise information-processing strategy. This strategy should, at least on relatively simple tasks, result in performance enhancements. However, if the tasks are perceived as a threat to self-esteem, then control-deprived individuals may protect their self-esteem by withdrawing effort and attributing their subsequent poor performance to a lack of effort (rather than to the more esteem-debilitating factor of lack of ability).

The Learned-Helplessness Model of Depression

In a major statement of his model of learned helplessness, Seligman (1975) has suggested that learned helplessness consists of three interrelated deficiencies: motivational, cognitive, and emotional. More specifically, Seligman has proposed that learned helplessness: "(1) reduces the motivation to control the outcome; (2) interferes with learning that responding controls the outcome; (3) produces fear for as long as the subject is uncertain of the uncontrollability of the outcome, and then produces depression" (Seligman, 1975, p. 56). Noting the similarities between these deficits produced by exposure to uncontrollable outcomes and those characteristic of depression in humans, Seligman (1975) also has suggested that learned helplessness may be viewed as a model of naturally occurring depression in humans. That is, just as learned helplessness is produced by exposure to uncontrollable outcomes (expectancy of response–outcome independence), reactive depression may also be caused by feelings of loss of control over behavioral outcomes, and may be accompanied by cognitive, emotional, and motivational deficits similar to those that accompany states of learned helplessness (i.e., symptoms of passivity, negative cognitive sets, and depressed affect). Accordingly, laboratory-induced helplessness should produce deficits parallel to those found in naturally occurring depression (Klein et al., 1976).

This learned-helplessness model of depression has stimulated an impressive amount of research (see the review by Garber, Miller, & Seaman,

1979). An early study reported by Klein et al. (1976) is representative of this research. In their study, Klein et al. assigned depressed and nondepressed college students to one of five training sessions during which they received (a) solvable problem, (b) no problems, (c) unsolvable problems with no-attribution-of-failure instructions, (d) unsolvable problems with internal-attribution-of-failure instructions, and (e) unsolvable problems with external-attribution-of-failure instructions. When subsequently tested on a series of anagrams, depressed students performed worse than nondepressed students and students who had received solvable or no-discrimination problems during the training session. Also, in accord with the learned-helplessness model of depression, subjects who received unsolvable problems during the training phase showed performance deficits parallel to those exhibited by depressed students. Finally, Klein et al. (1976) found that when depressed students were led to attribute their failure to the difficulty of the problems rather than to their own lack of ability, performance improved significantly. Klein et al. (1976) concluded:

The learned helplessness model of depression is strongly supported by our results: Laboratory-induced helplessness produced deficits parallel to those found in naturally occurring depression. In addition, however, the learned helplessness model of depression needs an extra construct concerning attribution of helplessness to personal failure. . . . Because all the early helplessness studies were done with animals, the early theory did not need knotty constructs like attribution and personal adequacy. Now that helplessness can be studied in man and because helplessness has been proposed as a model for human depression, learned helplessness theory now needs to incorporate such mediational cognitions (p. 516).

While the study by Klein et al. (1976) manipulated depressed individuals' causal ascriptions for their performance outcomes, a study by Kuiper (1978) examined depressives' and nondepressives' typical patterns of attributions for successful and unsuccessful outcomes. Specifically, in this study depressed and nondepressed college students performed a word association task and then received feedback indicating they had answered 20%, 55%, or 80% of the items correctly. Following task performance, students were asked to assign causal responsibility for their performance outcomes to effort, ability, task difficulty, and luck. The results indicated that nondepressives made internal attributions (ability, effort) for success and external attributions (task difficulty, luck) for failure. In accord with Klein et al.'s (1976) findings suggesting that learned helplessness is dependent upon exposure to failure *and* the attribution of helplessness to internal causes, Kuiper reported that depressives made internal attributions for failure. Contrary to expectations, depressives also made internal attributions for successful outcomes. In discussing these findings, Kuiper speculated that

nondepressives' external attributions for failure may represent an effective strategy (i.e., the operation of a self-protective bias) for preventing the occurrence of depression. On the other hand, the depressive's tendency to make a personal attribution for failure may be a very ineffectual strategy for preventing the occurrence of depression. . . . For instance, it is possible that blaming oneself for failure may contribute to other features of depression, such as feelings of unworthiness, guilt, self-devaluation, and loss of self-esteem (p. 243).

The results found by Klein et al. (1976) and Kuiper (1978), then, suggested that for humans causal attributions following uncontrollable outcomes may mediate subsequent performance deficits. These results, however, also raised questions about the learned-helplessness model of depression. For example, if depression results from a belief in response–outcome independence, why do individuals attribute causal responsibility for failure to themselves (Abramson & Sackheim, 1977)? Indeed, Abramson et al. (1978) noted that the original formulation of the learned-helplessness model of depression suffers from four major inadequacies:

(a) Expectation of uncontrollability per se is not sufficient for depressed *affect* since there are many outcomes in life that are uncontrollable but do not sadden us. Rather, only those uncontrollable outcomes in which the estimated probability of the occurrence of a desired outcome is low or the estimated probability of the occurrence of an aversive outcome is high are sufficient for depressed affect. (b) Lowered self-esteem, as a symptom of the syndrome of depression, is not explained. (c) The tendency of depressed people to make internal attributions for failure is not explained. (d) Variations in generality, chronicity, and intensity of depression are not explained (p. 65).

All but the first of these inadequacies have been addressed by Abramson et al. (1978) in a reformulation of human helplessness (see also Miller & Norman, 1979). It is to this reformulated model that we now turn our attention.

Reformulated Model of Learned Helplessness

According to the reformulated model of helplessness, the individual first learns that certain outcomes are not contingent on his or her responses. The individual then makes an attribution regarding this noncontingency of responses and outcomes to stable–unstable, internal–external, and global–specific causes. This causal attribution determines the individual's subsequent expectation for future noncontingency, and the expectation, in turn, determines the helplessness symptoms that result (i.e., the generality and chronicity of helplessness deficits, and lowered self-esteem). The sequence of events that, according to the reformulated model, lead to symptoms of helplessness are illustrated in Table 7.1.

To elucidate the role of attributions in the production of learned helplessness symptoms, Abramson et al. (1978), like other attribution theorists and researchers (e.g., Heider, 1958; Kelley, 1967; Weiner, 1974), have proposed that causal attributions can be classified along internal–external

TABLE 7.1. Sequence of events leading to helplessness symptoms (adapted from Abramson, Seligman, & Teasdale, 1978).

Perceived noncontingency	→ Attribution of noncontingency to factors that are a. stable–unstable b. global–specific c. internal–external	→ Expectation of future non-contingency	→ Helplessness symptoms a. chronic deficits b. general deficits c. lowered self-esteem

and stable–unstable dimensions. The internal–external dimension differentiates those causes that are due to some aspect of the person (e.g., ability or effort) and those that result from situational or environmental factors (e.g., task difficulty or luck). The stable–unstable dimension refers to factors that are long-lived and recurrent (e.g., ability or task difficulty) versus those that are short-lived and nonrecurrent (effort or luck). In their attributional reformulation of learned helplessness, Abramson et al. (1978) have argued that attributions may also be classified along a third dimension: global–specific. According to these authors global factors occur across situations and affect a wide variety of outcomes, whereas specific factors are unique to the learned-helplessness situation and do not generalize across situations.

What implications do attributions to internal–external, stable–unstable, and global–specific dimensions have for future expectations of noncontingency and symptoms of helplessness and depression? Abramson et al. (1978) have suggested that following a perception of noncontingency, attributions to internal factors lead to "personal helplessness" and depression (i.e., the person expects the outcome is not contingent on any response in his or her repertoire but that relevant others may have available the requisite response), while attributions to external factors lead to "universal helplessness" and depression (i.e., the person expects the outcome is not contingent on any response in his or her repertoire nor on any response in relevant others' repertoires). Moreover, attributions to internal factors are more likely to lead to self-esteem loss than attributions to external factors. In addition, attributions to stable factors should produce helplessness and depression deficits that are characterized by greater time-related characteristics than attributions to unstable factors. Finally, deficiencies attributed to global factors are more likely to generalized across situations than those attributed to specific factors.

Abramson et al. (1978) speculated that there may be a depressive attributional style. Specifically, these authors suggested that "the particular attribution that depressed people choose for failure is probably irrationally distorted toward global, stable, and external factors" (Abramson et al., 1978, p. 68).

Within the past decade, considerable research testing various aspects of the reformulated model has appeared (for reviews of this literature see Coyne & Gotlib, 1983; Peterson & Seligman, 1984; Sweeney, Anderson, & Bailey, 1986). The theoretical hypothesis that probably has received the most attention has been the existence of a depressogenic attributional style. Consider a prototypic study. Seligman et al. (1979) developed an attributional style questionnaire in which college students were asked to imagine themselves receiving positive and negative outcomes in various situations and to describe the major cause of the outcome. The students then were asked to rate that cause on the dimensions of internality, stability, and globality. Seligman et al. (1979) found that depressed students explained negative outcomes in terms of internal, stable, and global factors to a greater degree than did nondepressed students. Depressed student's attributions for positive outcomes were more external and unstable. In another study, Rapps, Peterson, Reinhard, Abramson, and Seligman (1982) found that depressed patients were more likely to attribute bad outcomes to internal, stable, and global causes than were nondepressed schizophrenic and nondepressed medical patients. These results, then, support the notion of a depressive attributional style that is not a general characteristic of psychopathology (see also Ingram, Kendall, Smith, Donnell, & Ronan, 1987).

While a number of studies have found evidence consistent with the notion of a depressive attributional style, it is important to note that a number of investigators have reported disconfirming findings (e.g., Hammen & Cochran, 1981; Hammen & DeMayo, 1982; Miller, Klee, & Norman, 1982). In an attempt to determine the strength of the depression–attribution relationship, Sweeney et al. (1986) recently conducted a statistical review of over 100 published studies. The evidence presented in this review on the whole strongly supports the attributional-style–depression hypothesis. Specifically, as attributions for negative outcomes become more internal, stable, and global, depression increases. While the reformulated learned-helplessness model of depression does not explicitly make predictions regarding causal attributions for positive outcomes, it does imply that attributions to internal, stable, and global factors ought to be negatively correlated with depression. Such a relationship was found by Sweeney et al. (1986) in their review of the evidence; however, the depression–attribution relationship for positive outcomes, while significant, was not as strong for positive as it was for negative outcomes.

Sweeney et al. (1986) also examined whether a number of possible factors suggested by authors in the literature affected or mediated the strength of the depression–attribution relationship. They found that for the most part, the type of subject (college student or psychiatric depressive), type of outcome (hypothetical or real), type of depression measure, and type of setting (classroom, laboratory, hospital) produced nonsignificant or weak and inconsistent effects.

This review of the available literature, then, provided relatively strong support for the depressive–attributional-style hypothesis. This is particularly noteworthy given the rather modest reliability (.4 to .7) of most questionnaires designed to assess attributional style (Peterson & Seligman, 1984). A new and expanded version of the most frequently used measure, the Attributional Style Questionnaire (Peterson et al. 1982), recently has been published (Peterson & Villanova, 1988) and holds the promise of permitting more satisfactory tests of the reformulated model.

Concluding Points

We have seen that attributions for outcomes, particularly negative outcomes, to internal, stable, and global factors are associated with depression (see also Brown & Seigel, 1988). A number of issues relevant to the learned-helplessness model of depression remain, however.

First, the model is quite specific regarding the nature of the depression–attribution association: The attributional style is thought to be a preceding, contributory cause of depression. Since most of the data reviewed by Sweeney et al. (1986) were correlational, they really do not address the direction-of-causality issue. What really is needed to assess the causal relationship between attributions and depression are longitudinal studies. The few longitudinal studies that do exist in this area do not yield uniformly supportive evidence. Golin, Sweeney, and Schaeffer (1981), Firth and Brewin (1982), Nolen-Hoeksema, Girgus, and Seligman (1986), and Seligman et al. (1984) provide evidence that at least some dimensions of the attributional style precede depression; other investigators (e.g., Cochran & Hammen, 1985), however, have reported disconfirming evidence. There are a number of methodological differences that might explain these inconsistent results (see the review by Barnett & Gotlib, 1988). Perhaps the most we can say at this point is that the causal role of attributions in depression has yet to be demonstrated conclusively.

Second, the unique components and consistency of a depressive attributional style have been questioned. Several investigators have noted that the attributional dimensions of internality, stability, and globality often are correlated (see chap. 2). Indeed, at least two researchers (Anderson & Arnoult, 1985) have argued that only two components—the controllability and locus dimensions—are involved in the depressive attributional style. Questions about the consistency of the style generally have to do with the cross-situational nature of the style. Anderson, Jennings, and Arnoult (1988) recently have provided evidence of the convergent and discriminant validity for attributional styles assessed at an intermediate level of specificity (i.e., they are specific to broad classes of situations).

Third, the origins of the depressive attributional style are not addressed by the helplessness model. However, research provides us with some clues (see Fincham & Cain, 1986, for a developmental analysis of learned helplessness). There is some evidence, for example, that attributional style may be learned directly or through modeling from parents (Seligman et al., 1984) or from differential feedback delivered by teachers in educational settings (Dweck & Licht, 1980). A final possibility is that the reality of individuals' first traumatic loss—the extent to which it actually is caused by internal, stable, and global factors—may set their attributional style for life (Peterson & Seligman, 1984).

Finally, we have discussed attributional style as it relates to depression. However, explanatory style has been shown to play a role in a variety of failures of adaptation, including loneliness (Anderson & Arnoult, 1985; Anderson, Horowitz, & French, 1983), shyness (Anderson & Arnoult, 1985), and low self-esteem (Tennen & Herzberger, 1987). Clearly, considerable theoretical and empirical work that indicates when one type of failure versus another will result is needed.

Attributional Processes and the Emotional Exacerbation of Dysfunctional Behaviors

In our preceding discussion of learned helplessness (Abramson et al., 1978), we examined how attributional processes may produce behavioral deficits and depression. Storms and McCaul (1976) also have proposed that attributional activities may lead to severe psychological disturbances. Specifically, these authors have suggested that under certain conditions, attributions to self may increase symptomatic behavior by triggering anxiety. Consider, for example, the insomniac who upon retiring begins to wonder whether this will be another sleepless night. Suddenly, our insomniac notices that it's a little warm and that the faucet in the bathroom is dripping. After tossing and turning for about an hour, it's still warm, the drip sound like Niagara Falls, and it's getting lighter outside. Our insomniac gets more anxious and begins to wonder if her inability to sleep is really a symptom of some more serious psychological problem. It even occurs to our insomniac that she may be neurotic and need long-term psychotherapy.

This pattern of behavior is characteristic of a number of different emotional syndromes. In such a pattern, the individual becomes aware of an undesirable aspect of his or her own behavior, such as insomnia. From that individual's point of view, the behavior is a symptom of some underlying problem, a lack of control, a basic inadequacy. These negative self-attributions produce further anxiety that, in turn, exacerbates the original symptomatic behavior.

Storms and McCaul (1976) have formulated an attributional model to account for the emotional exacerbation of dysfunctional behaviors. These authors have proposed that a self-attribution of unwanted, dysfunctional behavior results in an increased emotional state of anxiety and that this anxiety may serve to increase the frequency or intensity of the dysfunctional behavior. Storms and McCaul noted that their exacerbation model should be applicable to three general categories of maladaptive behaviors.

First, behaviors which are comprised of specific physiological functions may be disrupted by anxiety. This category would include sleeping, sexual functioning, and perhaps certain motor tasks that require precise muscular movements. Second, behaviors which are habitual, well-learned responses may be increased by anxiety. This category may include various addictions, alcoholism, over-eating, and perhaps other typical emotional responses to stressful situations. Third, behaviors which require attention to appropriate cues may be affected by anxiety. This category would include driving and other perceptual-motor tasks, and test taking and other highly cognitive activities (Storms & McCaul, 1976, p. 154).

In a test of their exacerbation model, Storms and McCaul (1975) examined the role of subjects' attributions about their speech disfluencies upon subsequent disfluency rates. More specifically, normal-speaking subjects were asked to make two tape recordings of their speech. After subjects completed the first recording, the experimenter informed all subjects that they had displayed a very high number of disfluencies such as repetitions and stammers. Next, half of the subjects were told that their disfluency rate was a normal result of situational factors such as being in an experiment; the remaining subjects were told that their disfluency was a symptom of their own, personal speech-pattern ability. All subjects then were asked to make the second tape under conditions of high or low situational stress (i.e., subjects were told that their second tape either would or would not be played with identifying information to a psychology class). Storms and McCaul predicted and found that self-attribution/high-stress subjects exhibited significantly greater increases in stammering than all other groups.

The results of this study provide support for the notion that the internalization of a negative self-attribution may lead to exacerbation of dysfunctional behavior. It is important to note, however, that the subjects in Storms and McCaul's (1975) test of their exacerbation model were normal-speaking subjects; they had no real speech problem. In addition, while Storms and McCaul were able to produce temporarily an increase in stammering in the self-attribution/high-stress subjects, we cannot assume that the same underlying process is responsible for an experimentally induced and a naturally occurring speech disorder.

In a more recent study, Lowery, Denny, and Storms (1979) applied the exacerbation model within the context of naturally occurring symptoms. Subjects in this study were insomniacs. Half of these subjects were assigned to a pill-treatment condition in which they received a placebo; these subjects were told that the "pill" would arouse them. Lowery et al. hypothesized that these subjects could reasonably attribute their insomnia to the pill and thereby avoid self-blame. The remaining subjects in this study were assigned to a self-attribution treatment group and were told that they were personally responsible for their failure to get to sleep, but that they should not worry. They further were shown bogus recordings of their physiological responses indicating that their arousal was elevated, but not abnormally high. The results of this study indicated that compared to no-treatment control subjects, the insomniacs in both treatment groups found it easier to get to sleep; interestingly, even subjects in the self-attribution group reported falling asleep more quickly.

This latter finding has important implications for the exacerbation model. It is possible that not all self-attributions for dysfunctional behaviors will result in an exacerbation of symptoms. If, for example, the attribution is to factors that, while internal to the individual, are also unstable and controllable, then the likely implication will be that the individual has the ability to change or prevent the symptomatic behavior (Janoff-Bulman, 1979). Alternatively, it may be possible, as Lowery et al. (1979) demonstrated, to reinterpret the magnitude of the emotional reaction accompanying negative self-attributions.

Concluding Points

In this chapter, we have examined attributional processes as they relate to Seligman's (e.g., Abramson et al., 1978) learned-helplessness model of depression and to Storms and McCaul's (1976) model of the emotional exacerbation of dysfunctional behaviors. Both models propose that causal attributions influence an individual's cognitive, affective, and emotional reactions to stressful life events. This emphasis on social–cognitive processes has stimulated a considerable amount of research on the development and maintenance of dysfunctional behaviors and has highlighted the necessity of placing psychopathology within its social context. In the next section, we will turn our attention from social–psychological processes involved in the development of problem behaviors to a discussion of research suggesting that under some conditions, invididuals may use existing symptoms, regardless of their origins, to protect esteem.

Symptoms as Self-Handicapping Strategies

In chapter 2, we discussed the well-documented tendency for individuals to take more causal credit for their successes than for their failures. This self-serving bias is one example of the use of attributions to protect and enhance esteem. Another is the proactive creation of multiple plausible causes of performance, some of which may serve as excuses for poor performance should it occur (for a review, see Arkin & Baumgardner, 1985, and Berglas, 1986. This use of attributional principles has been termed self-handicapping (Jones & Berglas, 1978), and relies on Kelley's (1972b) discounting and augmentation principles (see chap. 1). Basically, the self-handicapper, it is argued, reaches out for impediments, exaggerates handicaps, and embraces any factors that (a) permit discounting of the handicapper's actual ability as a cause for failure, or (b) augment the handicapper's ability as a cause for successful performance (in the face of plausible extraneous reasons).

An early study reported by Jones and Berglas (1978) demonstrates how self-handicapping works. In this study, presumably concerned with "the effects of drugs on intellectual performance," subjects were exposed either to contingent- (i.e., performance feedback followed subjects' attempts to offer solutions to soluble problems) or noncontingent- (i.e., performance feedback followed subjects' attempts to offer solutions to insoluble problems) success experiences. All subjects then were asked to choose between performance-inhibiting and performance-facilitating drugs whose effects would be active during a retest. The investigators reasoned that noncontingent-success individuals would lack confidence that their successful performance could be repeated and, consequently, would strategically choose situations where future success could be attributed by themselves and by others only to their personal characteristics. As predicted, males chose the performance-inhibiting drug significantly more often in the noncontingent-success condition than in the contingent-success conditions. For reasons that were not entirely clear, female subjects' drug choice was unaffected by the contingent or noncontingent nature of the success experience.

Since this initial study, handicapping via the acquisition or claim of a variety of internal but nonability-related handicaps, as well as external impediments to performance, has been reliably demonstrated (e.g., Greenberg, 1983; Kolditz & Arkin, 1982; Rhodewalt & Davison, 1984; Tucker, Vuchinich, & Sobell, 1981). While external impediments need not put the handicapper in a bad light, the same may not necessarily be true of internal handicaps such as taking a performance-debilitating drug, consuming alcohol, or withdrawing effort from some task. Still, such handicaps permit the avoidance of the more debilitating attribution of incompetence.

Will individuals go so far in their attempt to obscure the causal link between ability and poor performance as to use their symptoms of psychological problems as handicaps? The answer apparently is yes. Smith, Snyder, and Handelsman (1982) asked students who were high and low in trait anxiety to take an intelligence test, and they led these students to believe that scores on this test could (or could not) be affected by anxiety. These authors reasoned that highly test-anxious students would be more likely than low-test-anxious students to use their symptoms to create ambiguity about the causes of their negative outcomes and, consequently, would be more likely to report anxiety when anxiety was presented as a viable explanation for poor performance on the intelligence test. Smith et al.'s (1982) results supported these predictions. Moreover, when highly test-anxious subjects could not create ambiguity about the cause of their potentially negative outcomes via self-reports of anxiety, they did so by reporting less expenditure of effort on the test.

The use of symptoms as excuses for potential future failure has been examined within contexts other than test anxiety. Evidence also indicates that symptoms of depression, shyness, and hypochondriasis may be employed in a handicapping fashion (Baumgardner, Lake & Arkin, 1984; Smith, Snyder, & Perkins, 1983; Snyder, Smith, Augelli, & Ingram, 1985).

The notion that symptoms of psychological disorders may be used to excuse poor performance assumes that some audience, either the handicapper him/herself or others, believes that the symptoms should reasonably and legitimately reduce the handicapper's causal responsibility. The excuse value of psychopathological symptoms recently was investigated by Schouten and Handelsman (1987). Their subjects responded to a hypothetical case study describing either a male or a female protagonist in one of two situations: domestic violence or poor job performance. Additionally, subjects were told that the protagonist (a) currently displayed symptoms of depression, (b) currently displayed symptoms and had a history of psychiatric involvement, or (c) there was no mention of current or past symptomatology.

Schouten and Handelsman reported that depressive symptoms significantly reduced subjects' attributions of the protagonist's causal influence, responsibility, and blame for his or her behavior. Depressive symptoms also led generally to less punitive sanctions. Finally, the presence of a psychiatric history led subjects to hold lower standards for the protagonist's future behavior. These results, then, provide some support for the hypothesis that depression may be viewed as a legitimate excuse (see also Hill, Weary, & Williams, 1986) for undesirable behavior.

Concluding Points

While considerable research now demonstrates that individuals will use their psychological symptoms or other impediments to obscure the causal link between ability and poor performance, the motivation underlying this use of attributional principles is not entirely clear. We have argued here that self-handicapping serves to protect public (Kolditz & Arkin, 1982) and/or private (Berglas & Jones, 1978) esteem. It is important to note, however, that the research findings also are consistent with the notion that individuals will under certain conditions create causal ambiguity to preserve their behavioral control (Snyder & Wicklund, 1981). In addition to esteem-damaging implications, an attribution of poor performance to a lack of ability also would imply constraints on the range of future performance outcomes. The degree to which self-handicapping reflects control or esteem maintenance motivations is a question that can only be answered after additional theoretical and empirical work. Also important is the question of the factors that determine the selection of a handicap; in most, if not all, of the research in this area, subjects are given only one plausible handicap (a debilitating drug, effort withdrawal, psychological symptoms). Finally, the consequences, both public and private, of adopting a self-handicapping strategy deserve attention.

8
Attributional Processes, Treatment of Maladaptive Behaviors, and the Maintenance of Behavior Change

In the preceding chapter, we reviewed several current areas of research that illustrate the potential importance of attributional processes in the etiology and maintenance of various dysfunctional behavior patterns. This research in social and cognitive factors involved in the development and maintenance of maladaptive behaviors also has been accompanied by an increased interest in the incorporation of attribution principles to treatment procedures (e.g., Brewin & Antaki, 1987; Forsterling, 1985; Harvey & Galvin, 1984; Kopel & Arkowitz, 1975; Ross, Rodin, & Zimbardo, 1969; Valins & Nisbett, 1972). In an early paper, Valins and Nisbett (1971) attempted to describe how social-psychological research on attribution processes may be relevant to the area of clinical practice. Since the appearance of this paper, a number of researchers have investigated the application of attributional principles to the treatment of clinically important problem behaviors. In this chapter, we will examine both social-psychological and clinical research relevant to two major forms of attributional treatments of various maladaptive behaviors: misattribution and attributional-retraining therapies. We also will examine the empirical evidence regarding the possible relationship between a patient's attributions about his or her treatment improvements and the maintenance of his or her behavioral changes.

Aversive Emotional States and Misattribution Treatment Interventions

Misattribution of Source of Arousal

More often than not clients initiate or are referred for psychotherapeutic treatment because of distressing emotional states that are interfering with their daily functioning. It is not uncommon, for example, for individuals to seek treatment for anxiety that interferes with their sleeping, their performance on exams, or their ability to interact with strangers. Before considering how attribution processes may play a role in the treatment of such distressing emotional experiences, it is necessary to consider the possible role of causal attribution in the production of emotions.

As described in chapter 2, Schachter (1964) has proposed a theory of emotion which posits that both perceptible physiological arousal and labeling of this arousal in accord with situational or cognitive factors are necessary for the subjective experience of emotional stress. An attributional analysis of Schachter's theory suggests that diffuse physiological arousal motivates the individual to make causal attributions about the source of his or her autonomic arousal and that these causal attributions in turn provide the individual with cognitive labels (e.g., fear or anger) for the arousal state (Ross et al., 1969; Valins & Nisbett, 1971). According to this analysis, then, physiological arousal attributed to an emotionally relevant source should result in emotional behavior. The specific nature of this behavior would, of course, depend upon the nature of the cognitive label attached to the arousal state. However, physiological arousal attributed to a non-emotional source should not result in emotional behavior.

This attributional analysis of Schachter's (1964) emotion theory has stimulated a considerable amount of research. Much of this research has attempted to demonstrate that undesirable emotional behaviors (in particular, defensive behaviors) may be reduced by leading individuals to misattribute their heightened autonomic arousal to nonemotional sources.

In an early study designed to test this misattribution of arousal notion, Nisbett and Schachter (1966) attempted to persuade subjects that physiological arousal accompanying fear of electrical shocks was actually produced by a nonemotional source. Specifically, these investigators told subjects they would receive either a series of mild electrical shocks (low-fear condition) or a series of painful electrical shocks (high-fear condition. Prior to receiving the shocks, all subjects were given a placebo pill and a description of physiological reactions alleged to be side effects of the drug. For one half of the subjects, the description of side effects included physiological symptoms characteristic of fear, while for the remaining subjects the description of side effects included physiological symptoms irrelevant to fear.

As predicted, subjects in the low-fear condition who were led to believe their physiological arousal was due to the drug (i.e., those subjects who were given descriptions of fear-relevant side effects) found the shocks less painful and tolerated higher shock intensities than did low-fear condition subjects who were led correctly to attribute their arousal to the electrical shocks. Moreover, a postexperimental questionnaire indicated that the attribution manipulation was successful with low-fear subjects. In contrast to subjects in the low-fear conditions, Nisbett and Schachter (1966) reported that high-fear subjects did not differ in their reports of pain or tolerances of electrical shock as a function of the attribution manipulation.

Further, the postexperimental questionnaire revealed that the attribution manipulation was not successful for subjects in the high-fear conditions. That is, most of these subjects attributed their heightened physiological arousal to the electrical shocks, regardless of the drug or shock-attribution instructions. The investigators had expected that their attribution of arousal manipulation would not be effective for high-fear subjects since the anticipation of painful electrical shocks would be too plausible an explanation for their arousal.

While Nisbett and Schachter's study demonstrated that subjects could be verbally persuaded to misattribute their arousal to a nonemotional source and subsequently to display a reduction in emotional (i.e., defensive) behavior, it also suggested that misattribution might be possible only "within the limits of plausibility." Specifically, the results of this study indicate that misattribution of arousal might not be possible when individuals have a salient and plausible explanation (e.g., painful electrical shocks) for their extreme emotional responses.

Recognizing that this limitation could greatly limit the potential application of misattribution procedures in clinical settings, Ross et al. (1969) conducted a study designed to serve "as an experimental analogue to plausible therapeutic techniques" (p. 279). Ross et al. reasoned that for highly fearful individuals, misattribution procedures might be more effective if the correlation, or causal connection, between the emotionally relevant source and physiological arousal were obscured. In this study, subjects were told that the purpose of the experiment was to determine the effects of distracting noise on task performance. The task required subjects to learn to assemble two puzzles. Subjects were told that the solution of one of the puzzles would lead to monetary reward, while the solution of the other puzzle would allow them to avoid an electrical shock. In fact, both puzzles were insoluble. Next, all subjects were informed that the noise to which they would be exposed during task performance might have side ects. Half the subjects were led to believe that they would experience side effects which correspond to the usual physiological correlates of fear (e.g., palpitations). The remaining subjects were led to believe that they would experience side effects which are not usually associated with fear but which could be associated with noise bombardment (e.g., ringing sensation in the ears). These experimental instructions were intended to induce subjects to attribute their physiological arousal state (produced by the anticipation of receiving painful electrical shocks) either to the threat of shock or to a cognitively neutral source (i.e., noise bombardment), and they consistently were presented contiguous with the onset of arousal symptoms. Finally, subjects were presented with the two puzzles and allowed to spend as much of the available test period working on each puzzle as they wished.

Ross et al. reasoned that the greater fear of shock would be reflected by more time spent on the shock-avoidance puzzle. Moreover, higher levels of fear should be exhibited by shock-attribution subjects who were not given the opportunity to misattribute their physiological arousal to the cognitively neutral source. In accord with predictions, the results of this study indicated that shock-attribution subjects spent significantly more time attempting to solve the shock-avoidance puzzle than did noise-attribution subjects.

Ross et al.'s (1969) study, then, demonstrated that even for highly fearful individuals, avoidance behaviors could be reduced through attribution techniques. The generalizability to clinical settings of the results of this study, as well as those reported by Nisbett and Schachter (1966), is questionable, however, since neither of these studies used clinically relevant target behaviors nor clinical problems.

Clinical Applications

A first attempt at testing the implications of misattribution-therapy techniques for a clinically important problem was provided by Storms and Nisbett (1970). Before describing the Storms and Nisbett investigation, let us consider a real-world example that may illuminate different aspects of the misattribution process depicted by these investigators. Suppose a student becomes extremely anxious before taking exams and consults a clinician about this problem. One possible treatment might be some type of tranquilizing drug. Another possibility might be to give the student an extremely mild tranquilizer or a placebo but to tell the student that the drug will lead to a very high level of relaxation. The question arises: During the next exam, will the student, who may feel some anxiety, think about the clinician's description of the effects of the drug and become *less* anxious? Or will the student think that the presumably strong drug was unable to relieve this anxiety and, therefore, become *more* anxious (i.e., will the student think that if he or she is anxious despite the medication, then his or her anxiety must be very severe)?

In an attempt to answer such questions, Storms and Nisbett asked insomniacs to take a placebo pill a few minutes before going to bed. Subjects were told either that the pill would produce physiological symptoms characteristic of arousal (e.g., alertness, palpitation, high body temperature) or that the pill would produce physiological symptoms characteristic of relaxation (e.g., relaxation, lowered heart rate, decreased body temperature). The authors reasoned, "to the extent that an insomniac goes to bed in a state of autonomic arousal and associates that arousal with cognitions that are emotionally toned, he or she should become more emotional and have greater difficulty getting to sleep" (1970, p. 320). However, if an insomniac is led to attribute part of his or her arousal at bedtime to a drug, he or she should experience less emotionality and, consequently, get to sleep sooner. In accord with these predictions, Storms and Nisbett (1970) found that insomniacs anticipating drug effects characteristic of arousal reported getting to sleep more quickly on nights they took the pills. Also as predicted, insomniacs expecting drug effects characteristic of relaxation reported getting to sleep less quickly on nights they took the pills, presumably because they assumed that their emotional responses must have been extremely intense to have counteracted the effects of the relaxation pill.

Storms and Nisbett's (1970) study, then, has obvious clinical relevance. It suggests that if a client's problems are exacerbated by anxiety over symptoms, providing the client with a nonemotional source for his or her physiological arousal will reduce maladaptive emotional behavior. However promising Storms and Nisbett's results appear for clinical applications of misattribution techniques, it is important to note that the results obtained by these investigators have been diffcult to replicate. For example, studies reported by Kellogg and Baron (1975) and Bootzin, Herman, and Nicassio (1976) found direct-suggestion, or placebo, effects rather than the reverse placebo effect obtained by Storms and Nisbett. That is, in both of these studies insomniacs given drug-arousal instructions identical to those used by Storms and Nisbett (1970) reported an increase in time to fall asleep. Because of these failures to replicate the results reported by Storms and Nisbett and because of the sole reliance on self-report measures of latency to fall asleep in the Storms and Nisbett (1970), Kellogg and Baron (1975), and Bootzin et al. (1976) studies (as well as the Lowery et al., 1979, study reported in chapter 7), the clinical potential of misattribution techniques with insomniac clients remains somewhat controversial.

In a conceptual replication of Storms and Nisbett's (1970) design, Singerman, Borkovec, and Baron (1976) examined the effects of misattribution of arousal manipulations on another clinically relevant problem, speech anxiety. These investigators asked highly and moderately anxious speech-phobic subjects to present two speeches. During the presentation of the speech, subjects were exposed to meaningless noise in a manner similar to the procedures employed by Ross et al. (1969). Subjects were told either that the noise bombardment was known to increase physiological arousal (arousal condition) or that it was known to suppress or eliminate physiological arousal (sedation condition). In addition, all subjects were informed that their speeches would be videotaped for later evaluation and that an observer would be rating their performances during the speech presentations.

The results reported by Singerman et al. (1976) failed to replicate the misattribution effects found by Storms and Nisbett (1970), Ross et al. (1969), and Nisbett and Schachter (1966). Consistent with the findings reported by Kellogg and Baron (1975) and Bootzin et al. (1976), the results of self-report and behavioral measures of anxiety indicated direct placebo or suggestion effects; when noise was present, arousal subjects exhibited slightly and nonsignificantly more anxiety than did sedation subjects. Singerman et al. (1976) noted that the failure to replicate misattribution of arousal effects was likely due to the failure of their attribution manipulation. Most subjects attributed their heightened physiological reactions to anxiety about public speaking regardless of the arousal or sedation instructions.

It is important to note that this failure of the attribution manipulation in the Singerman et al. (1976) study is entirely consistent with Schachter's (1964) theoretical statement and with experimental results reported by Nisbett and Schachter (1966). Schachter (1964) stated, "given a state of physiological arousal for which an individual has no immediate explanation, he will 'label' this state and describe his feelings in terms of the cognitions available to him" (p. 53). However, if the individual has a ready explanation for his or her arousal, then he or she will be unlikely to search for alternative causal explanations. In the Singerman et al. (1976) study, it seems reasonable to argue that subjects had an immediate and salient causal explanation for their arousal. That is, the salience of anxiety caused by speech presentations may have been exaggerated by the experimenters' emphases on (a) taping subjects' speeches for later evaluation, and (b) observers' ratings of subjects' performances. It is not surprising, then, that subjects labeled their arousal as caused by the speech situation.

Shyness is another problematic behavior pattern that has been addressed via the misattribution logic. Brodt and Zimbardo (1981) placed shy and not-shy females in an interactive situation with a male confederate. Prior to the interaction, subjects were exposed to loud noise. Subjects were told that the noise would produce a pounding heart and increased pulse rate. It was assumed that the shy women would attribute their interaction anxiety to the noise and thereby be less anxious. A physiological record of subjects' pulse rates showed that the shy women experienced a decrease in pulse rate from pretest levels (a reverse placebo effect), whereas the not-shy women manifested an increased in pulse rate (a standard placebo effect).

Expectancy-Attribution Model of Placebo Effects

While this brief examination of the literature indicates that misattribution of arousal techniques sometimes alleviates nonclinical target behaviors and clinically relevant problems, it also reveals a number of studies in which misattribution predictions have not been supported (see also Cotton, 1981; Reisenzein, 1983). Ross and Olson (1981) have presented an expectancy-attribution model of the effects of placebos in an attempt to resolve the inconsistencies in the literature. Their model outlines a number of conditions that are necessary for misattribution to occur: (a) the cause of arousal must not be obvious; (b) the misattribution source should be salient; (c) subjects must believe that the misattribution source is a plausible cause of their arousal (e.g., the onset of arousal must be contiguous with the onset of the misattribution source); and (d) subjects must believe that the misattribution source is producing more extreme effects than it really is.

The model also distinguishes primary assessments, which measure the direct effects of the expectancies associated with the placebo, from secondary assessments, which measure the recipient's inferences about underlying dispositions that are not believed to be directly affected by the placebo (inductive effects). In addition, placebos whose presumed impact will counteract the recipient's symtoms (conunteractive expectancies) are distinguished from placebos whose presumed effects will parallel the recipient's symptoms (parallel expectancies). According to the model, standard placebo effects are expected on primary assessments of counteractive-expectancies placebos. Reverse inductive effects (altered inferences about an underlying disposition in the direction opposite to the placebo's alleged impact) are likely on secondary assessments of parallel-expectancies placebos. Consider, for instance, what happens when recipients of parallel-expectancy placebos attempt to gauge the severity of their underlying condition from examination of their symptoms. The expectancy-attribution model predicts that if individuals exaggerate the effect the placebo had on their symptoms (i.e., they believe their symptoms are caused by the placebo), then they are likely to underestimate the degree to which symptoms are caused by their underlying condition. Consequently, they may believe that their underlying condition is less severe than they would have believed it to be had the placebo not been administered (reverse inductive effects).

Ross and Olson's (1981) expectancy-attribution model is theoretically compelling and promises to bring order to an important but chaotic literature. Support for their model of placebo effects has been found in several studies (e.g., Olson & Ross, in press; White & Kight, 1984). It is important to note, however, that a reasonable, alternative interpretation exists for these and many other misattribution studies. Leventhal and his associates (Calvert-Boyanowski & Leventhal, 1975; Leventhal, Brown, Shacham, & Engquist, 1979) have argued that the reduction of emotional reactivity or distress typically found in misattribution studies might have been due not to the emotional relabeling of bodily states, but to the mere presentation of veridical arousal information. More specifically, these authors have noted that in most of the misattribution studies, a major difference between arousal and sedation subjects has been the receipt of veridical arousal information by the former and the receipt of nonveridical arousal information by the latter. Thus, any observed reductions in emotional behavior by the arousal subjects might have resulted from the congruence between their expectations of physiological reactions and their actual experience.

While it is clear that veridical preparatory information about physiological reactions does affect emotional behaviors, a recent study reported by Olson (1988) supported the misattribution argument that decreases in emotionality (in this case, speech anxiety) are due to causal inferences regarding the source of arousal, not to the presentation of accurate information alone. Clearly, some theoretical integration of the preparatory information and misattribution models will be necessary to identify the conditions under which one or the other is applicable.

Concluding Points

From this examination of the misattribution-of-source-of-arousal literature, what conclusions can be drawn regarding the therapeutic potential of
misattribution-of-arousal techniques? Several studies (e.g., Nisbett and
Schachter, 1966; Singerman et al., 1976) suggest that it may be difficult to
manipulate attributions about the source of arousal with certain clinical
problems, such as phobias, where the emotional response is clearly associated with a salient explanation. With such clinical cases, the more extreme
and/or chronic the emotional response, the more difficult it probably would
be to manipulate the client's belief about the source of arousal. Often,
however, the source of a client's distress may not be apparent or may become more ambiguous during the course of treatment. Consider, for example, the college student who initiates treatment because she is experiencing considerable anxiety associated with reduction of cigarette smoking. In
this case, the source of the college student's anxiety may seem obvious.
However, during the course of treatment, she also discloses that she is
anxious about graduating from college, about not having a job, and about
her boyfriend interviewing for jobs in another state. As a result, the clinician may be able to effect a reduction in her level of anxiety by persuading
her to attribute her arousal to some relatively neutral source. In psychologically ambiguous conditions, then, misattribution techniques may be
effective in reducing arousal regardless of the intensity or chronicity of the
emotional state (Fincham, 1983b).

   Several authors have dismissed the therapeutic potential of misattribution of arousal techniques (e.g., Bandura, 1977). While such an extreme
position may be premature, the use of misattribution techniques does present certain problems for practitioners. They do, for example, entail some
amount of deception, and for ethical reasons many practitioners may
reject them (Storms, Denney, McCaul, & Lowery, 1979). Some of the
reattribution-training techniques to be discussed later in this chapter do not
have the problems nor the potential limits (e.g., Ross & Olson's, 1981,
preconditions) on their use that the misattribution-of-arousal approaches
may have. Before examining the reattribution-training literature, however,
we need to discuss briefly a variant of misattribution therapy.

Misattribution of Degree of Arousal

According to Schachter's (1964) theory of emotions, both perceptible physiological arousal and labeling of this arousal in accord with situational or
cognitive factors is necessary for the subjective experience of emotional
states. In the preceding section, we examined studies that investigated the
possibility of manipulating individuals' beliefs about the source of their
heightened physiological arousal. The possibility that actual autonomic
arousal may not be necessary for the production of emotional responses as
long as individuals *believe* they are aroused has been investigated in a series

of studies conducted by Valins and his associates (Valins, 1966; Valins & Ray, 1967).

In the studies of greatest clinical interest, Valins and Ray (1967) suggested that the reduction of avoidant behaviors produced by systematic desensitization might be dependent upon the manipulation of cognitions about internal reactions to the phobic stimulus. These investigators had unselected subjects (study I) randomly view 10 slides of snakes and 10 slides of the word "shock." In addition, presentations of the shock slides were followed by single administrations of mild electrical shocks. While viewing the slides, experimental subjects heard what they believed to be their heart rate increase in response to the shock but not to the snake slides. Control subjects heard the same sound as did the experimental subjects but were told that they were meaningless sounds. Valins and Ray reasoned that to the extent experimental subjects believe they are no longer affected by the phobic stimulus (i.e., slides of snakes), they also will believe they are no longer afraid of snakes and will exhibit more approach behavior when subsequently exposed to a live snake. The obtained results supported this hypothesis; experimental subjects approached and held a live snake more often than did control subjects. It is important to note, however, that this effect was statistically significant only after subjects who had previously touched a snake were excluded from the analyses.

Valins and Ray (1967) conducted a second study in order to examine whether manipulation of cognitions regarding internal responses would affect avoidance behaviors in subjects whose fear of snakes was more extreme. Specifically, in this second study Valins and Ray recruited subjects who reported on a preexperimental questionnaire that they were afraid of snakes. The procedure for this second study was identical to that used in the first, with two exceptions. First, subjects viewed through a one-way mirror a live snake in a glass cage instead of the slides of snakes. Second, in place of the conventional behavioral-avoidance task used in the first study (and in most studies of systematic desensitization), Valins and Ray (1967) used the amount of money required to induce subjects to touch a snake as a measure of snake-avoidance. This task was used because Valins and Ray felt the conventional task might be too frightening for subjects whose fear of snakes was relatively intense. Consistent with the results of the first study, the experimental subjects, led to believe that they were not aroused following exposure to the caged snake, required less pressure (i.e., less money) to touch the live snake than did control subjects.

Valins and Ray's (1967) studies of the effects of "cognitive desensitization," or the misattribution of the level of arousal, suggest that persuading a client to believe that he or she is no longer afraid of a phobic stimulus is sufficient to reduce avoidant behaviors. A number of investigators, however, have criticized the therapy-analogue procedure employed by Valins and Ray in their studies. More specifically, the results reported by Valins and Ray have been called into question because (a) a relatively weak behavioral posttest was used in study II (Bandura, 1969); (b) a behavioral pretest of fear associated with snakes was not employed, and such pretests typically eliminate a large number of subjects who report fear on a screening questionnaire (Gaupp, Stern, & Galbraith, 1972; Kent, Wilson, & Nelson, 1972; Sushinsky & Bootzin, 1970); (c) the obtained behavioral effects might have been due to differential attention paid by experimental subjects to their supposed heartbeats (Stern, Botto, & Herrick, 1972); and (d) an aversion–relief model (i.e., a procedure whereby two stimuli are randomly presented, and one of the stimuli is followed by an electrical shock while the other is followed by no aversive consequence and thus takes on reinforcing properties) could account for the obtained group differences in avoidance behavior (Gaupp et al., 1972; Stern et al., 1972). More importantly, the results reported by Valins and Ray (1967) have been difficult to replicate.

An experiment reported by Conger, Conger, and Brehm (1976) attempted to address several of the issues noted above. These authors argued that failures to replicate the results of Valins and Ray (1967) may have occurred for two possible reasons:

Subjects in the replication studies were generally more fearful than those in the original study, and the use of a behavior pretest may have mitigated the effect of false heart-rate feedback (Conger et al., 1976, p. 135).

In their study, Conger et al. examined the proposition that fear level may be a moderator of the effect of false-heart-rate feedback. Specifically, subjects whose fear of snakes was relatively high or low were assigned to noise or false-heart-rate-feedback conditions. The experimental procedure used in the Conger et al. study was nearly identical to that employed by Valins and Ray (1967). In addition to investigating the effects of fear level, these investigators varied the contiguity between shock and snake slides in order to provide a direct test of the aversion–relief explanation of Valins and Ray's results. As predicted, low-fear subjects in the feedback condition exhibited more approach behavior toward a live snake than low-fear subjects in the noise condition. However, high-fear subjects showed no effects on the behavioral posttest as a function of feedback versus noise conditions. Conger et al. (1976) also found no support for the aversion–relief explanation of the effects of false-heart-rate feedback on avoidance behavior.

Conger et al. (1976), then, demonstrated that fear level is a critical factor in the replication of Valins and Ray's (1967) results; that is, reduction in avoidance behaviors via manipulation of cognitions about internal reactions was evident only for subjects whose fear of snakes was relatively low. The finding that behavioral effects resulting from misattribution of degree of physiological arousal and difficult to obtain with high-fear subjects is consistent with Schachter's (1964) theory of emotion and with the conclusions drawn earlier regarding misattribution-of-source-of-arousal studies (e.g., Nisbett & Schachter, 1966; Ross & Olson, 1981). Some degree of psychological ambiguity concerning either the source of heightened arousal or the level of physiological arousal seems to be necessary in order to manipulate attributions and the labeling of emotional states. Thus, when a highly fearful individual experiences a salient and intense internal reaction in response to a fear-relevant stimulus, it would probably be difficult to modify his or her interpretation about the level of the internal response.

Such a conclusion is clearly disappointing in terms of the clinical potential of misattribution-of-degree-of-arousal procedures. The level of fear (or other distressing emotional states) experienced by many clients is likely to make the use of such procedures difficult. Moreover, ambiguity with respect to the source of arousal is more likely to exist or to be more easily created in clinical populations than ambiguity concerning the degree of internal reactions. Perhaps because of these concerns about the clinical potential of misattribution-of-degree-of-arousal procedures, there have been very few studies examining their use in the past decade.

Attribution-Retraining Treatment Interventions

In the preceding sections of this chapter, we examined studies relevant to the possibility of a misattribution therapy, an intervention whereby the adoption of a new attribution for arousal symptoms might result in the lessening of undesirable effects of those symptoms. In this section, we will examine another variant of attributional approaches to behavior change, attribution retraining. This attributional approach to behavior change is concerned not with altering attributions regarding physiological arousal but, rather, with altering an individual's "attributional style" in response to specific aversive events.

Before examining studies relevant to attribution-retraining interventions, it is necessary to note that the area of behavior change recently has seen a proliferation of treatment strategies (Bandura, 1977), such as rational–emotive therapy (Ellis, 1962) and cognitive–behavior modification (e.g., Meichenbaum, 1977; Rehm, 1981), that emphasize the importance of cognitive processes as mediators of behavior change. Moreover, many of these cognitively based treatment interventions examine aspects of a client's cognitions or "internal dialogues" other than self-attributions (e.g., self-appraisal, expectancy, competence, self-reinforcement.) Several of these treatment approaches appear to have considerable clinical potential and have stimulated a good deal of research. However, here we will focus only on studies designed to investigate the possibility that attributional styles may be modified and that such modifications may result in more adaptive behavioral patterns. We should note that most of the research concerned with the modification of attributional styles has occurred within the context of achievement behaviors; we will postpone discussion of this important research until chapter 9.

Attribution Retraining and Depressive Attributional Styles

In chapter 7, we examined in some detail the reformulated learned-helplessness model of depression. This model asserts that helplessness depression results when individuals expect that they will not be able to exert control over and attain the goals they desire and consider important. In addition, these individuals will show a loss of self-esteem when they believe that relevant others, unlike themselves, can exert control and reach these goals. Beach, Abramson, and Levine (1981) assert that four points of treatment intervention for a depressive episode derive from the reformulated model:

(1) Reverse people's expectations that they have no control over important goals; (2) facilitate a change from unrealistic to more realistic goals; (3) decrease the importance of unattainable goals; and (4) when appropriate, reverse people's expectations that other people do have control the important goal, whereas the person does not (i.e., change an internal attribution for uncontrollability into an external attribution) (p. 124).

It is this latter point that we will focus on in our discussion. While the notion of a depressive attributional style (i.e., the tendency to make internal, stable, and global attributions for uncontrollable, aversive outcomes) as a risk factor for depression has generated a good deal of research, until very recently there have been few attributional-change studies guided by this notion (Forsterling, 1985).

In one of these, Peterson and Seligman (1981) content-analyzed verbatim transcripts of initial, middle, and termination psychotherapy sessions with depressed patients. Transcripts were rated in terms of the internality, stability, and globality of explanations spontaneously offered for life events entailing a loss. Peterson and Seligman reported that explanatory style perfectly ordered the three sessions for each patient; the most internal, stable, and global explanations were offered during the initial sessions, and the least internal, stable, and global attributions were offered during the last session.

These results have been supplemented in a more recent investigation (Seligman et al., 1988). Seligman et al. administered to 39 depressed patients the original Attributional Style Questionnaire (ASQ) (Seligman et al., 1979), as well as the Beck Depression Inventory (BDI) (Beck & Beck, 1972), at the beginning and end of cognitive therapy (Beck, Rush, Shaw, & Emery, 1979) and at a one-year follow-up session. As predicted, analyses revealed a positive correlation between ASQ and BDI scores; at intake, termination, and follow-up more internal, stable, and global explanations for bad events were related to more severe depressive symptoms. Additionally, explanatory style and severity of depression improved dramatically and in lockstep fashion with one anothr during the course of cognitive therapy. Moreover, these improvements were maintained at the one-year follow-up session.

These results raise the possibility that modification of explanatory style may be the active therapeutic ingredient in cognitive therapy for depression (Seligman, 1980). It is important to note, however, that both the Peterson and Seligman (1981) and Seligman et al. (1988) studies of attribution-style change during psychotherapy are correlational in nature. It is possible that explanatory-style change was a result rather than a consequence of successful cognitive therapy (cf. Peterson, Luborsky, & Seligman, 1983). As Seligman et al. (1988) note, it will be necessary for future research to examine session-by-session changes in explanatory style, depressive symptoms, and therapeutic content to examine the causal role of attributional retraining in alleviating depression.

Attribution Retraining and Locus of Control

The notion that attributional explanations for negative life events presented during psychotherapy can have beneficial effects, while not tested directly in depression research, has been examined in the social-anxiety literature. In one study, for example, Forsyth and Forsyth (1982) had trained counselors administer therapy to individuals who had identified themselves as interpersonally anxious and desirous of treatment for their anxiety. During the course of "causal counseling," clients were exposed to one of two interpretations for their interpersonal difficulties. One of these emphasized that social anxiety, though stemming from internal factors, was controllable (internal/controllable-counseling condition); the other noted that many people experience social anxiety, but that socially skilled persons have learned to cope with this nervousness (coping-counseling condition). The results of this study indicated that both attributional treatments were effective in reducing clients' levels of social anxiety. However, the attributional interpretations were differentially effective depending on clients' locus-of-control orientations (Rotter, 1966). Specifically, the more internal the client, the more he or she benefitted from the internal/controllable-causal treatment. Additionally, there was a tendency for the coping treatment to be less effective for internal clients.

Concluding Points

The results of research on attribution retraining reviewed here, as well as additional work (e.g., Altmaier, Leary, forsyth, & Ansel, 1979; Baumgardner, Heppner & Arkin, 1986; Johnson, Ross, & Mastria, 1977) tentatively suggest that exploration of the causes of stressful events can have therapeutic effects. In addition to replicating and extending these findings, however, a number of important issues remain. It will be important to examine whether attribution treatments are more effective for some target behaviors than others. It also will be necessary to investigate the most effective methods of modifiying attributional styles (Forsterling, 1985).

Finally, considerable conceptual and empirical work will be needed to specify what specific causal interpretations for what kinds of problems will be most effective for which clients (Forsyth & Forsyth, 1983).

Attributions for Treatment Gains and the Maintenance of Behavior Change

That causal attributions may be implicit in treatment interventions is forcefully illustrated in the following interview excerpts presented by Whalen and Henker (1976) in their examination of attitudinal and cognitive correlates of Ritalin administration. These comments of an 11-year-old demonstrate how positive behavior change can be attributed to medication and, in addition, how misbehavior can be attributed to nonmedication:

Child: Well, sometimes I go in the bedroom and start crying because I need it, you know. And then my mother will come in and ask me what's wrong, and I'll say, "Daddy won't let me take my pill." She'll say, "Come on down here—I'll give it to you." So, I'll go down and she'll give it to me."
Interviewer: So, sometimes you can really tell that you need it.
Child: Yeah. [Pause] Sometimes I get mad at my dog and if I start getting mad at my dog, my Mother will say, "Go take your pill." I'll say, "Ah—O.K.," and I'll go downstairs and take it and then I come back upstairs and start saying "I'm sorry" to my dog.
[Later]
Child: At school two boys that know karate are gonna teach me how to do it. If I don't take my pill I'll start doing it on them (1976, p. 1126).

Several other authors also have acknowledged the possible attributions that may follow from various treatment procedures and have stressed the importance of such attributions in maintaining positive behavioral change (e.g., Bandura, 1977; Brehm, 1976; Meichenbaum, 1977; Valins & Nisbett, 1972). For example, Bandura, Jeffrey, and Gajdos (1975) have stated:

Attributional processes may similarly delimit gains from success experiences. When disinhibition is facilitated by extensive supports, people may ascribe their success to external aids rather than to their own restored capabilities. Generalization decrements are more likely to occur if bold performances are attributed to special situational arrangements, rather than to regained personal competence (p. 142).

An early study by Davison and Valins (1969) examined the possibility that behavior change attributed to oneself would persist or be maintained to a greater degree than behavior change attributed to an external agent such as a drug. Subjects in Davison and Valins's "experimental analogue of drug therapy" (a) received a series of shocks and indicated their pain thresholds and shock tolerances, (b) ingested a pill (actually a placebo), (c) repeated the series of shocks with shock intensities surreptitiously halved by the experimenter, and (d) again indicated their pain thresholds and tolerances. Because the experimenter had reduced the shock intensities, all subjects presumably were led to believe that the drug had improved their threshold performances. Next, half of the subjects were told they had been given a placebo, while the other half were given no such information. In a third series of shocks, it was found that subjects who attributed their behavior change to themselves (i.e., those who believed they had ingested a placebo) tolerated more shock and perceived the shocks as less painful than did subjects who attributed their behavior change to the drug. These results suggest that if an individual attributes positive behavior change to medications, and consequently does not feel responsible for the behavioral improvement, he or she is unlikely to maintain the change once medication is stopped. However, if an individual attributes positive behavioral changes to himself or herself, such changes are more likely to persevere.

A study by Davison, Tsujimoto, and Glaros (1973) also examined the generalization of treatment gains as a function of attributions about the causes of such gains. However, this study may be more relevant to clinical settings than the Davison and Valins (1969) study since Davison et al. were concerned with a clinically relevant target behavior, insomnia. In this study, insomniacs participated in a week-long treatment program consisting of pharmacological procedures (self-produced relaxation and scheduling of evening activities prior to going to bed). Following treatment, half the subjects were told that they had received an optimal dosage of the sleeping aid, while the others were told they had received a dosage that was too weak to have been responsible for any improvement. Following this attributional manipulation, all subjects were asked to discontinue the drug but to continue the relaxation and scheduling procedures for an additional week.

The results indicated that both optimal and minimal dosage groups showed equivalent and significant treatment effects; subjects in both conditions reported shorter latencies to sleep in the treatment than in the baseline weeks. Moreover, greater maintenance of treatment gain during the posttreatment week was demonstrated by subjects who could not attribute their improvement to the drug. These results offer support for the notion that behavioral changes believed to be due to an external agent, like a drug, generalize less to the posttreatment situation than changes believed to be due to one's own effort. However, the posttreatment period employed by Davison et al. (1973) was very short. It is possible that the generalization effects dissipated over time. There are, however, several more recent studies that demonstrate an association between self-attributions for behavioral change and long-term maintenance (for example, see the discussion of Colletti and Kopel, 1979, in chap. 9).

The study by Davison et al. (1973) appears to provide meaningful support for the role of self-attributions as predictors of maintenance of behavior change. Additional support has been found in studies examining the maintenance of health-related treatment gains such as weight reduction (Jeffrey, 1974; Sonne & Janoff, 1979), alcoholism (Davies, 1982), and smoking cessation (Colletti & Kopel, 1979). Also, several authors (e.g., Bandura, 1977; Brehm, 1976; Valins & Nisbett, 1972) have noted that induction of desired attributions for treatment gains need not involve deceptive manipulations. For example, internal attributions for behavioral improvements may be induced by gradually reducing and eliminating external aids once a client is performing the desired behaviors.

Concluding Points

In conclusion, attribution therapies have been enjoying increasing popularity in the modification of maladaptive behavior patterns and in the maintenance of treatment gains. While the evidence indicates that misattribution and attribution-retraining treatment interventions may be useful therapeutic procedures, it also suggests that under certain conditions misattribution regarding the source and level of physiological arousal may be difficult to achieve. In particular, research indicates that it may be difficult to manipulate attributions about the level and/or source of arousal with certain clinical problems, such as phobias, where the emotional response is clearly associated with a salient explanation. Future research will need to assess for which clinical disorders attribution therapies are effective. In addition, investigators will need to assess the clinical utility of research findings relevant to attributional processes and the treatment of maladaptive behaviors. While treatment gains may be statistically significant, the clinical significance of such gains will need to be determined before actual treatment programs based upon attributional principles are developed.

9
Attributions and Achievement

The nature of attributions within educational settings has been the focus of a significant amount of research within the attribution literature. Because evaluation is such an integral part of our educational system, it is important to understand how students react to the feedback they receive about their schoolwork. Perceptions of whether they have succeeded or failed academically, along with analyses of why their performance was rated as such, can have a significant impact on expectancies for future performance, mood, and subsequent academic behavior. This chapter will review literature which describes the type of attributions students typically make following academic success or failure. The impact of these attributions on expectancies, mood, and future behavior also will be examined. Finally, literature will be reviewed which suggests that attributions can be modified in an attempt to improve future academic performance.

In general, the articles reviewed here will address the nature and impact of students' attributions for their own academic performance rather than teachers' attributions of pupils' performances. Although the achievement–attribution literature has had widespread application, space limitations preclude examination of topics such as the impact of labels (e.g., mental retardation) on attributions for academic performances (e.g., Bromfield, Weisz, & Messer, 1986) and the nature of attributions in various cross-cultural populations (e.g., Graham & Long, 1986; Powers & Wagner, 1983). (For additional reviews of the achievement–attribution literature, the interested reader is referred to Forsyth, 1986, and Weiner, 1986.)

Attributions Following Academic Success or Failure

The search for attributions within the realm of achievement behavior typically has involved questions regarding the reasons for success or failure at some academic task (e.g., a set of math problems, a course exam, a semester grade). The majority of the literature within this domain has examined attributions of academic outcomes to four primary causes: ability, effort, luck, and task difficulty. Use of these causes was based on Heider's early statements regarding the nature of attributions (see chap. 1), although Weiner and his colleagues (see Weiner, 1974; Weiner et al., 1971) were leaders in establishing the centrality of these causes within the domain of achievement behavior. As the reader will see below, Weiner et al.'s focus on the internal/external and "can"/"trying" components of attributions reflected the strong impact of Heider's writings on their work.

In the early experimental analyses of attribution–achievement links, subjects imagined or experienced academic success or failure and subsequently evaluated the cause of the outcome in terms of ability, effort, luck, and task difficulty (e.g., Frieze & Weiner, 1971). In subsequent work, however, subjects were given the chance to respond more freely. For example, at times they were asked more generally, "Why did the outcome occur?" While data from these subsequent studies substantiated the notion that attributions to ability, effort, luck, and task difficulty were common and spontaneous responses (e.g., Frieze, 1976; Frieze & Snyder, 1980), additional causes such as mood, value of the outcome, and the behavior of others were cited as important (Elig & Frieze, 1979; Forsyth & McMillan, 1982; Frieze, 1976).

Weiner's Early Formulation

In an early analysis of achievement attributions, Weiner et al. (1971) hypothesized that people inferred causality about academic success or failure on the basis of perceptions about an individual's ability to complete the task in question, the degree of effort expended, the difficulty of the task, and the degree to which luck influenced the outcome. Weiner et al. (1971) also proposed that these causes varied along two primary dimensions: locus of control and stability. The locus of control dimension (see chap. 1) concerned the degree to which a cause was related to factors within the person (internal cause) or the external environment (external cause). Internal causes included both ability and effort attributions (the "can" and "trying" components described by Heider), whereas external causes included variables such as luck and task difficulty. It was noted by Weiner et al. (1971) that both internal and external causes could fluctuate across time as well as situations. For example, although ability and effort are both internal variables, ability is typically perceived to be a relatively enduring personal characteristic whereas effort fluctuates more easily over time and across situations. In addition, one usually thinks of luck as an external, changeable cause whereas task difficulty is perceived as a less variable aspect of the environment. This categorization scheme proposed by Weiner et al. (1971) is presented in Table 9.1.

TABLE 9.1. Categorization of achievement-related causes along dimensions of stability and locus of control (adapted from Weiner, Frieze, Kukla, Reed, Rest, & Rosenbaum, 1971).

	Stability	
Locus of control	Stable	Unstable
Internal	Ability	Effort
External	Task difficulty	Luck

Empirical Data Addressing Weiner's Conception

Some consistencies have emerged across laboratories with regard to the typical pattern of attributions reported following academic success and failure. In particular, a number of studies reported that attributions to internal causes were more likely to occur following successful academic outcomes, whereas external causes were more likely to be called upon to explain academic failures (Bernstein, Stephan, & Davis, 1979; Frieze & Weiner, 1971; Kovenglioglu & Greenhaus, 1978). In these studies, college subjects who did well on a course exam (or who imagined themselves or others doing well) were more likely to endorse attributions such as ability and effort than students who perceived their own or others' behavior as a failure. On the other hand, students who failed (or imagined themselves or others failing) emphasized bad luck or the difficulty of the test as being important causes for the outcome.

Data from at least two additional studies suggested that stability of causes, in addition to locus of control, was an important aspect of attributions following academic success and failure. First, Arkin and Maruyama (1979) reported that following actual performance on a college exam, students were more likely to attribute perceived success (relative to perceived failure) to both internal and stable causes. Second, stability was an important variable in a study conducted by Frieze (1976). In this study college subjects were given the opportunity to provide their own explanations of imagined academic outcomes in a free-response format (i.e., they were not asked only to rate the importance of causes provided for them by the experimenters). Analysis of free responses demonstrated that success was attributed more often than failure to ability (an internal, stable cause), whereas failure was attributed more often to being in a bad mood (an internal, unstable cause). Here, stability appeared to be a more important attributional dimension than locus of control in differentiating causes for success and failure.

The importance of the stability dimension will become further evident in the next section of this chapter when we analyze the relationship between attributions and expectancies for future performance. However, the data reviewed to date suggest that a bias may exist for attributing successful academic performances to internal and probably stable causes while attributing academic failures to external (and perhaps unstable) causes. This pattern is reminiscent of the self-serving attributional biases described in chapter 2. Possible explanations for this pattern were discussed in that chapter and will not be reiterated here.

Individual Differences

Early research in the achievement–attribution domain included consideration of individual differences in subjects' achievement motivation or needs for achievement. These individual-difference variables had been a central focus in general achievement literature since the early 1960s (e.g., Atkinson, 1964). As psychologists developed interests in attributions, it became of interest to discover whether individuals characterized as low or high in need for achievement demonstrated different attributional patterns following academic performances. As reviewed by Weiner (1986), early studies suggested that subjects high in achievement needs showed a stronger self-serving bias for failure than individuals low in achievement needs (e.g., Meyer, 1970). In other words, high need for achievement was associated with ascribing failure to lack of effort (internal, unstable) while low need for achievement was associated with attributing failure to lack of ability (internal, stable). Other data suggested that high-need achievers attributed success to high ability and effort and failure to lack of effort, whereas low-need achievers attributed failure to low ability and showed no clear preferences in attributions for success (e.g., Weiner, Heckhausen, Meyer, & Cook, 1972).

More recent work moved away from this focus on need for achievement. As Weiner (1986) noted, this movement resulted partially from difficulties in obtaining reliable measures of achievement motivation along with failures to replicate the findings reviewed above. Although some researchers continued to examine the relationships between achievement needs and attributions (e.g., Powers, Douglas, Cool, & Gose, 1985; Tepper & Powers, 1984), recent individual-difference work has focused more heavily on personality variations in attributional style. For example, individuals may have characteristic patterns of making attributions about their own and others' performances that are consistent across situations. This focus on attributional style will be noted subsequently when the work of Dweck and colleagues is discussed (e.g., Diener & Dweck, 1978, 1980; Dweck, 1975).

Concluding Points

Examination of attributional patterns following academic success or failure has focused on four primary causes—ability, effort, task difficulty, and luck—that vary along two major dimensions—locus of control and stability. Empirical data suggested that self-serving attributional patterns occurred frequently in achievement settings, such that successful academic outcomes were attributed to internal and/or stable causes while academic failures were attributed to external and/or unstable causes. As discussed in chapter 2, these attributional patterns may serve to enhance or maintain self-esteem, or they may result from differential modes of cognitive processing. It also appears that individual differences in achievement motivation may have some impact on attributional patterns in academic settings, although more recent personality approaches have moved toward consideration of individual differences in attributional style (see subsequent discussions of work by Dweck and colleagues).

Attributions and Expectancies for Future Performance

Given that we have some notions about the types of attributions made following academic success or failure, it becomes important to investigate the impact that these attributions have on various aspects of achievement functioning. The first such area to be reviewed concerns the relationship between attributions and expectancies for future performance—that is, how will perceptions of the causes for past performance influence what one expects to achieve in the future?

Research paradigms designed to investigate this relationship have taken one of two forms. First, correlational designs were used wherein subjects were asked to rate both attributions for a previous outcome and expectancies for a specific future performance. These ratings were made either following experience with some laboratory task in which success or failure was induced or after receipt of real-life academic feedback (e.g., an exam grade). The strength of statistical correlations between attributions and expectancies then served to estimate real relationships between the two concepts. Second, other studies manipulated causal attributions experimentally by telling subjects that certain outcomes occurred because of specified causes. The impact of these induced attributions on subjects' expectancies for future performance then were assessed.

Early Formulations

Weiner (1979, 1985, 1986) proposed that the stability dimension of attributions was central to assessing their impact on expectancies for future outcomes. If causes of past outcomes were perceived as remaining stable over time, expectations of future outcomes should be consistent with past outcomes—that is, "I got a good grade in the past because of my ability, and I expect my level of ability to remain constant over time. Therefore, in the future I expect that on similar tasks I also will perform well." Conversely, if causes are perceived as being unstable (i.e., fluctuating over time), individuals will not necessarily expect similar outcomes to recur.

Weiner's theoretical statement opposed an earlier, social-learning perspective proposed by Rotter (1966). Rotter's theory asserted the central importance of locus of control in moderating the impact of attributions on expectancies for future performance. Rotter contended that attributing past performance to internal causes should lead to increases in expectancies for success following successful outcomes or decreases in such expectancies following failure (these were named "typical expectancy shifts"). Alternately, attributing past performance to external causes was proposed to lead to "atypical expectancy shifts," or expectations of future outcomes opposite in nature from previous outcomes. Weiner contended that because Rotter typically investigated differential effects of attributions to ability and luck, dimensions of locus and stability were confounded. Specifically, ability can be categorized not only as an internal attribution but also as a stable one, and luck can be characterized both as external and unstable. Weiner further asserted that stability, rather than locus, had the major causal influence on expectancies. He and others provided empirical data to support this assertion.

Empirical Support for Early Formulations

In an early study by Weiner et al. (1972), German high-school subjects were exposed to repeated failure experiences with a digit-symbol substitution task. These students then were asked to attribute their performances to ability, effort, luck, or task difficulty, and were asked to provide subjective ratings of the probability that they would succeed on future digit-symbol task trials. Correlational analyses demonstrated that expectancies for future success were higher if subjects attributed their past failure to effort and luck (unstable causes) rather than to ability or task difficulty (stable causes). In other words, if John failed in the past due to a cause that varied over time, he was likely to believe that he had a better chance of succeeding on the next trial than if he attributed his past failure to something modifiable.

Bailey, Helm, and Gladstone (1975) also provided support for this relationship. In their study, college students attributed their performance on a midterm exam to one of the four basic causes and rated their confidence in obtaining a higher, lower, or similar grade on subsequent exams. Again, correlational analyses indicated a tendency for expectancies of future performance to be higher following failure if the failure was attributed to insufficient effort (unstable) rather than deficient ability (stable). (In the Bailey et al. study, however, stability was not significantly related to expectancies for success following past successful outcomes.)

Weiner, Nierenberg, and Goldstein (1976) conducted an additional study in this realm that has been cited as a crucial investigation in discriminating between the positions taken by Rotter (1966) and Weiner (1979). In this study, college subjects were given from zero to five success experiences with a modified-block-design task. They then made attributions for their performance and rated the number of subsequent trials they expected to solve correctly. Attribution measures in this study were designed to assess the impact of the four levels of attributional dimensions under investigation (stable/unstable, internal/external). Specifically, a separate set of ratings was made within each of these levels, such that one level remained constant while the other varied. Correlations indicated that expectancy for future success was highest when attributions were made to stable rather than unstable causes. This relationship occurred regardless of the level of the locus dimension specified (internal or external) and regardless of the number of success trials experienced by subjects. Overall, expectancy of success was not related significantly to the locus dimension. Hence, the data clearly supported Weiner's attributional perspective rather than Rotter's social-learning conception.

A study by Kovenglioglu and Greenhaus (1978) utilized a similar paradigm, but assessed the responses of college students who had just received a grade on a chemistry test. For subjects who perceived their past performance to have been a success, estimates of grades expected on a subsequent exam were significantly related to attributions of the previous grade to ability (internal, stable attribution). When subjects perceived their past grade as a failure, expectancies for future exam performance were significantly related to attributions of past grade to effort (internal, unstable attribution).

These data suggested that stability was a central characteristic of attributions that moderated their impact on expectancies for future performance. Weiner (1985, 1986) reviewed numerous additional studies that provided further support for this notion. Although these studies will not be described here, the interested reader is referred to Weiner's recent book on attribution and emotion (1986).

Theoretical Modifications

In addition to the controversy regarding the centrality of locus and stability dimensions in the relationship between attributions and expectancies, other dimensions were proposed as important in the attribution–achievement literature. In particular, following Kelley's early statements regarding the utility of attributions in establishing a sense of control (see chap. 1), Weiner (1979) proposed that controllability was a third central dimension to be considered in the achievement domain. Specifically, he noted that within each of the cells in Table 9.1 variability in the nature of a cause could occur based on the extent to which the cause was perceived as being within an individual's control. For example, mood and effort both could be classified as internal and unstable, but mood typically is perceived as being outside an individual's control whereas effort is seen as being personally controllable. Hence, controllability was proposed as a third important dimension in the analysis of attributions and achievement behavior.

Some empirical data substantiated the notion that controllability may moderate the impact of attributions on expectancies for future success. Forsyth and McMillan (1981a) assessed college subjects following receipt of exam feedback. Subjects attributed their performance to internal or external, stable or unstable, and controllable or uncontrollable causes (items were worded using these dimension terms rather than the more typical specific-causal terms). Subjects also evaluated, on a 9-point scale, how well they expected to do on future tests in the same class. Results indicated that stability of attributions had no significant relationship to expectancies. Rather, locus and controllability of attributions were related to expectancies such that failure attributed to external, uncontrollable causes was related significantly to low expectancies for future performance while success attributed to internal, controllable causes was related significantly to high expectancies for subsequent test grades. In other words, expectancy for future success was high if subjects believed that performance was due to a factor over which they themselves had some control. On the other hand, if performance was determined by some factor outside the subjects' control, expectancies for success were low. Forsyth and McMillan (1981a) cited a number of possible reasons for the divergence between their own and others' data, the most plausible of which was the failure of previous work to investigate the controllability dimension. Although data from a single study cannot be considered conclusive, these data certainly suggested that the impact of controllability of causes warrants further attention in this literature.

Other authors proposed even additional dimensions that may be important to a complete understanding of attribution–achievement relationships. Namely, globality of a cause (Abramson et al., 1978) and intentionality associated with an individual's behavior (Rosenbaum, 1972) have been cited as important. Even further dimensions have been proposed and were reviewed by Forsyth (1986). These will not be reiterated here, but it appears that further work will be necessary to analyze completely the dimensional structure of attributions (see chap. 2). However, as the list of dimensions becomes more extensive, it will be important to verify the relative importance of each dimension within various domains of functioning.

Concluding Points

The most consistent finding within the literature relating attributions and expectations for future academic performance has been the notion that stability of causes plays a central role. In a number of investigations, students expected future performance to be consistent with past performance when the latter was attributed to stable causes. Conversely, future performance was expected to be inconsistent with past performance when the latter was attributed to unstable causes. Location of causes for past performance along an internal/external dimension was not as important in influencing expectations, although more recent data suggested that other dimensions, in particular controllability, may be important to consider when examining the attribution–expectation relationship.

Attribution/Affect Links

As indicated earlier, attributions of academic success and failure have been linked not only to expectancies for future performance, but also to affective reactions. Following receipt of information that one has performed well or poorly on some academic task, a student may experience one or many of a variety of affective reactions such as pride or shame, happiness or sadness, and low or high self-esteem. In the past 15 to 20 years, a number of researchers attempted to examine the relationships between various attributions of academic performance and subsequent affective reactions.

Examination of the relationship between academic performance and affects such as pride or shame had a long history within the achievement-motivation literature (e.g., Atkinson, 1964). In the early 1970s, however, Weiner (1974) attempted to specify the role that attributions played in moderating this relationship. As should be recalled, within the domain of expectancies for future performance, considerations of the stability of causes appeared central in the majority of studies (although recent evidence suggested that controllability might be more important). In consideration of relationships between attribution and affect, however, it will become apparent that locus of control may play a more central role.

Weiner's Early Theoretical Position

Weiner's (1974) initial proposal suggested that internal attributions, relative to external attributions, should enhance pride or shame following academic success or failure. Specifically, if academic success were attributed to high ability or to hard work (internal attributions), a student should feel prouder of his/her accomplishments and should receive more external praise than if successful outcomes were attributed to external causes such as ease of the task or good luck. In addition, failure attributed to internal causes (e.g., low ability, insufficient effort expended) should lead to greater feelings of shame than failure attributed to external causes (e.g., difficulty of the test or bad luck).

These notions fit with the self-serving-bias interpretations of attributional patterns mentioned above and described in chapter 2. They also are intuitively appealing since one clearly should feel prouder of receiving an "A" on a term paper when one believes the grade was due to one's ability to write well or to extensive effort expended rather than to the fact that the assignment was an easy one or that the teacher gave an "A" to almost every student. Likewise, one is likely to feel more shame if a failing grade is perceived to be the result of an inability to comprehend the subject matter or lack of effort expended on the project than if the assignment were extremely difficult and everyone else in the class performed poorly. Due to the intuitive appeal of these ideas, as well as the convergence between them and available empirical data, the centrality of internal attributions for moderating the affect–academic-performance relationship was relatively well-accepted by other researchers.

A further proposition of Weiner's (1974) theory, however, was not as intuitively compelling, nor was it as well-accepted by other researchers in the field. Weiner maintained that within the domain of internal attributions, attributions to effort should have a stronger relationship with affective reactions than ability attributions. This proposition was based on data from Weiner and Kukla (1970). In this study, college and high-school subjects played the role of teachers and were asked to provide feedback for pupils whose performance on an exam was characterized by the experimenters in terms of ability and effort. Results indicated that rewards and punishment allocated by the teacher subjects for the pupils' performance were related more closely to what the subjects had been told about the levels of pupils' effort rather than information about their ability. In addition, subjects estimated that the pupils' pride in their success would be greatest when they exerted high effort and that shame following failure would be augmented given an attribution to low effort. Thus, Weiner and Kukla (1970) concluded that effort was of greater importance than ability in determining affective reactions in achievement situations.

Weiner (1977) subsequently extended these findings, suggesting that effort also should be more important in determining evaluation of an affective reaction to one's own experience with success or failure. In other words, I should feel prouder of an "A" on a test that I attributed to trying hard than an "A" that resulted from my ability to understand the subject matter. Similarly, I should feel more shameful of an "F" that resulted from lack of trying than an "F" due to lack of ability. Data from Brown and Weiner (1984) provided some support for this position. In this study, college students were asked to imagine succeeding or failing a required course. Subjects reported greater pride when success was attributed to high effort rather than high ability and greater shame when failure was attributed to low effort rather than low ability.

Alternate Theoretical Positions

Although most researchers agreed that internal attributions should have the greatest impact on affect following achievement behavior, the centrality of effort attributions was challenged by numerous researchers (e.g., Covington & Omelich, 1979a, 1979b; Nicholls, 1975, 1976; Sohn, 1977). The primary arguments centered around the relative importance of ability and effort attributions in determining affect. While some authors argued for the centrality of ability attributions (e.g., Covington & Omelich, 1979a,

1979b), others argued a moderate position wherein the impact of ability and effort attributions on affect depended on situational variables as well as the nature of the affect under investigation (e.g., Nicholls, 1975, 1976; Sohn, 1977).

Nicholls (1975, 1976) apparently initiated the ability/effort debate (Brown & Weiner, 1984). In an initial study, Nicholls (1975) reported that the level of pleasure subjects felt following academic success was more strongly associated with ability than with effort attributions. In a second study (Nicholls, 1976), subjects reported a preference to be judged as having high ability rather than high effort. Both of these papers called into question Weiner's position regarding the centrality of effort attributions. However, in the latter study (Nicholls, 1976), when the affect under consideration was pride or shame (rather than general feelings of pleasure such as those assessed in the initial study), the data were in line with Weiner's theory. In particular, pride and shame were more strongly associated with effort attributions than with ability attributions.

Sohn (1977) pursued these ideas further and found that, in accord with Weiner's theory, effort attributions were more important than ability attributions in determining feelings of pride and shame. Further, in accord with Nicholls' (1975) data, Sohn (1977) reported that ability attributions were more influential than effort attributions in determining unhappiness following failure. However, ability attributions were not more influential than effort attributions in determining general happiness following success. Sohn's (1977) only explanation for this latter pattern was that subjects had difficulty imagining themselves receiving an "A" due to significant ability. No manipulation checks were included, however, to substantiate such an explanation. Regardless, the data taken together (Nicholls, 1975, 1976; Sohn, 1977) indicated that the relationship between affective reactions and attributions was likely to vary depending on the type of affect under consideration.

Covington and Omelich (1979a, 1979b) took a less moderate position in critiquing Weiner's theory, arguing for the centrality of ability attributions in determining affect. Their argument was based on self-worth theory (Beery, 1975, Covington & Beery, 1976), which maintained that individuals are motivated to uphold perceptions of high ability in order to protect feelings of self-worth. In a recent paper, Covington and Omelich (1984) reviewed correlational data from an earlier unpublished study that supported their hypothesis. In that study, judgments of ability in a sample of college students were more strongly related to perceptions of self-worth than were perceptions of level of effort expended.

In earlier work, Covington and Omelich (1979a, 1979b) asked subjects to imagine succeeding or failing a test under conditions of high or low effort. Following imagined failure, both shame and dissatisfaction were associated with attributions to high effort (e.g., I tried very hard; I failed; I feel dissatisfied and shameful). Similarly, following success both pride and satisfaction were associated with attributions to effort (e.g., I tried hard; I succeeded; I feel proud and satisfied). The authors argued that the effort–affect relationships were moderated by attributions to ability. Specifically, attribution of failure to high effort maximized shame because of the implication that such attribution had regarding ability. For example, if I failed even though I tried very hard, I must have virtually no ability to perform well, and therefore I feel quite dissatisfied and shameful.

Some controversy continues to exist between the theories posited by Weiner (Brown & Weiner, 1984; Weiner & Brown 1984) and Covington and Omelich (1984), although Brown and Weiner (1984) argued that methodological differences may explain divergent empirical results. In particular, differences in subjects' ratings of the importance of achieving a certain outcome, variations in the content and wording of information provided to subjects to encourage certain attributions, and differences in the definitions of affective states under investigation occurred across studies (Brown & Weiner, 1984). With regard to the latter point, in Covington and Omelich's work public shame was investigated, whereas in Brown and Weiner (1984) guilt was examined. Empirical data from both groups suggested that public shame involves a sense of humiliation, which probably is influenced by ability attributions (Brown & Weiner, 1984; Covington & Omelich, 1979a, 1979b), whereas private shame appears to approximate more closely a feeling of guilt, which is associated with effort attributions (Brown & Weiner, 1984; Nicholls, 1975, 1976; Sohn, 1977).

Modifications of Weiner's Original Hypotheses

Critiques of Weiner's original theory contributed to modification of his position and the development of a more complete theory of attribution/affect linkages (Weiner, 1977, 1980, 1985, 1986). First, Weiner (1977) acknowledged that there was no reason to restrict an investigation of the affective consequences of attribution to evaluations of pride or shame. Second, he acknowledged that internal attributions (and effort attributions in particular) need not augment *all* affective states that occur following achievement outcomes. Rather, some affective states may be augmented by internal attributions while others may be intensified by external attributions. These modifications precipitated a more general search for attribution–affect linkages within research paradigms that assessed a *variety* of affective states.

In a series of studies, Weiner and colleagues (Weiner, Russell, & Lerman, 1978, 1979) demonstrated that a number of affective reactions were evoked following academic success or failure regardless of the nature of the attributions made. These reactions—happiness, satisfaction, confidence, depression, disappointment, disgust, and upset—were designated as outcome-dependent affects since they were influenced only by overall outcome (success or failure). These general reactions were the most intensely experienced emotions related to achievement behavior (Weiner, 1980), but other affective reactions were found to occur as a result of attributions to specific causes. In particular, ability attributions were associated with feelings of competence, pride, and resignation, while effort attributions were associated with feelings of relief, activation, and guilt. When performance was attributed to others, feelings such as gratitude or aggression were elicited, and outcomes attributed to luck elicited feelings of surprise.

Numerous reports (Bailey et al., 1975; Forsyth & McMillan, 1981a, 1981b; Kelley & Forsyth, 1984; McMillan & Forsyth, 1983) supported Weiner's notion that achievement outcome, regardless of attributions made, correlated significantly with general affective reactions following academic performance. Only weaker evidence exists, however, to support the existence of specific attribution–affect links. McMillan and Forsyth (1983), for example, assessed college students following receipt of an exam grade. Results indicated a large outcome-dependent effect on affect, and only weaker, specific links between the following: (a) effort attributions and ratings of performance value, (b) attributions to the course textbook or test characteristics and relaxation, surprise, competence, and contentment, and (c) attributions to luck and surprise reactions. When students were reassessed 1 week later, relationships between outcome and affective states remained significant, but significant relationships between causal attributions and affect were no longer apparent. These data suggested that any affective states which can be linked to specific attributions may be only temporary, and are certainly less stable than outcome-dependent affects.

A somewhat larger body of work focused less on the link between specific attributions and affective states and more on the relationship between affect and the general dimensions of attributions (e.g., locus, stability, and controllability). Weiner (1985, 1986) incorporated these ideas into more recent accounts of his theoretical position. In these, Weiner (1985, 1986) offered a description of a sequential process linking attributional thinking to emotional experience. As stated earlier, he suggested that following an achievement outcome, a general positive or negative emotional reaction occurs based on the perception that one has succeeded or failed. Perception of success or failure also initiates a search for causes of the performance outcome. Once appropriate causes have been identified, they then are located in dimensional space, being characterized as internal/external, stable/unstable, and controllable/uncontrollable. The dimensional properties of attributions then have psychological consequences that influence expectancies for future performance and create dimension-related affective states (as well as dimension-related expectancies and behavior, reviewed in other sections of this chapter).

In the dimensional conception, Weiner retained his earlier position that internal attributions should be linked to feelings of pride and shame. He added, however, the prediction that the controllability dimension should be linked to feelings of anger, gratitude, guilt, and pity, whereas the stability dimension should be associated with feelings of hopelessness/hopefulness (Weiner, 1985, 1986). As will be noted in the subsequent discussions, however, dimension–affect relationships are not consistent across studies.

As noted above, although controversy still exists regarding the centrality of specific attributions within the locus dimension (Covington & Omelich, 1979a, 1979b; Sohn, 1977; Weiner et al., 1978, 1979), all camps acknowledged the importance of examining the impact of internal versus external attributions on affect. As Weiner et al. (1978, 1979) reported, external attributions following successful test performance were associated with gratitude, surprise, and thankfulness, whereas internal attributions under the same conditions were related to feelings of pride, confidence, and satisfaction. Following failure, however, external attributions were related to feelings of anger, surprise, and hostility while internal attributions were associated with guilt, regret, and aimlessness. Although these data were collected in analogue or retrospective-recall paradigms, other data collected with college students following performance on a "real-life" exam support the importance of the locus of attributions in moderating emotional reactions (Arkin & Maruyama, 1979). Specifically, following receipt of an exam grade that students perceived as successful, internal attributions were associated with positive evaluations of the teacher and the course. Following perceived failure on the exam, external attributions were correlated with increased anxiety regarding the test situation. In this study, there also was support for the importance of stability of causes in influencing affect. Specifically, students who attributed their successful grade on the exam to stable causes felt less anxious about the test situation. For these subjects, the locus dimension of attributions had no effect.

Data from McMillian and Forsyth (1983) supported Arkin and Maruyama's (1979) position that stability of attributions moderates affect reported by college students following test performance. These researchers also reported that internality/externality of attributions was not as important as previous data had indicated. Rather, McMillan and Forsyth (1983) reported that stability and controllability dimensions were associated more strongly with emotional reactions than location of the attributions along a locus dimension. In this study, however, outcome itself (regardless of attribution) was the strongest predictor of reported emotion.

The importance of perceived controllability of causes in influencing affective states was reviewed by Weiner (1985). First, negative outcomes attributed to factors controllable by others elicit blame attributions, and usually are associated with anger reactions (Averill, 1982, 1983). For example, if an individual (person 1) receives a poor grade on a group project due to another student's careless work (person 2), person 1 is likely to feel anger toward person 2. Second, negative outcomes perceived to be the result of factors controllable by oneself are likely to lead to self-blame and feelings of guilt (Weiner, Graham, & Chandler, 1982). For instance, if a student believes that a poor grade on a test occurred as a result of factors that he/she could have controlled (e.g., not studying hard enough, not looking up additional information in the library), some type of guilt reaction is likely to result. Third, negative events attributed to uncontrollable factors seem to evoke feelings of pity (Weiner et al., 1982), and finally, gratitude is experienced when a positive event is attributed to factors that are perceived as controllable by others.

Forsyth and McMillan (1981a) added further evidence to support the claim that controllability of attributions is related to affect. In this study, although outcome was a primary predictor of general affect following exam feedback, controllability of the outcome also had a significant relationship with affect. Specifically, on 11 of 16 measures of affect, perceptions that outcomes were controllable were associated with more positive emotions than were perceived uncontrollable outcomes. Locus of attributions had only a slight effect on emotions. Overall, the most positive affect was reported by subjects who attributed successful academic performance (good exam grades) to controllable, internal, and stable factors.

Kelley and Forsyth (1984) reported further support for a dimensional relationship between emotion and attribution. These authors reported a significant outcome–emotion relationship, but also found that both affective reactions and attributions seemed to cluster into groups and that these groups were significantly related to one another. In particular, positive affective reactions were associated with attributions to facilitating personal factors (e.g., high motivation, good study habits, and adequate preparation) and instructional factors (e.g., good teaching methods, textbook, and class atmosphere). Negative affective reactions, on the other hand, were related to inhibiting factors (e.g., faulty teaching, inadequate preparation, poor test and text, low motivation, and personal problems).

Concluding Points

The data reviewed in this section supported Weiner's most recent position that outcome-dependent emotions occur in achievement situations and that these emotions often are experienced more strongly than other affective reactions. However, the data also suggested that Weiner's notions about the relationships between attributional activity and affective reactions have some validity. Strongest support was available for the position that specific affective reactions are associated with general dimensions of attributional activity rather than with specific causes. Nevertheless, there remains uncertainty regarding the precise nature of these relationships. It is likely that variables such as task importance, situational characteristics, and individual differences in achievement motivation or attributional style have some impact on attribution–affect linkages and that these links will not be persistent and stable across all conditions.

Attributions and Achievement Behavior

Attributions have been linked not only to expectancies regarding future performance and affective reactions following academic tasks, but also to actual performance on subsequent academic tasks. Specifically, attributions about past academic performance can influence the types of problem-solving strategies chosen for future tasks, the amount of persistence exhibited on difficult problems, and the accuracy of solutions to various types of problems. For example, if a student attributes his grade on a recent exam to the effort he expended in studying, he may be more likely to expend further effort in studying for the second test (to ensure a repeat performance) than if he believes he got a good grade just because the teacher likes him. In the latter case, one might believe it useless to expend effort to study if one probably will get a good grade regardless of the amount of studying. In accordance with data reviewed earlier, there also is evidence that individuals differing in degree of need for achievement may exhibit varying attributional patterns in achievement situations. These patterns in turn may influence academic performance (Weiner, 1986). However, also as reviewed earlier, the relationship between achievement motivation and attribution has been far from consistent across studies.

Early Empirical Work

In order to examine the impact of attributions on subsequent behavior in a real-life academic situation, Bernstein et al. (1979) assessed college subjects before and after three major exams in a semester-long psychology course. Subjects who attributed their performance on the first test to stable causes such as ability and ease of the test were more likely than other students to get a lower grade on the subsequent test. It may have been that when stable causes were perceived as responsible for past test performance, students studied less or in a less efficient manner given that they believed such effort would have little impact on their subsequent grade. Given that attributions to stable causes can lead to high expectancies for success, students may have felt no need to study. In addition, subjects who believed their third test grade would be related to the amount of effort they expended prior to taking it tended to get higher grades on the third test. When attributions to effort, therefore, became a more prominent explanation for expected test performance, grades improved.

Data from a study by Weiner et al. (1972) also suggested that attribution of past failure to stable causes such as deficient ability or difficulty of the task led to deterioration in subsequent performance. Other empirical work, however, has provided contradictory data. For example, Koven-glioglu and Greenhaus (1978) reported a significant relationship between ability attributions for current academic success and future exam performance. Students who believed they had done well on a test due to their own skill tended to get better grades on a subsequent exam. For these subjects, effort attributions for success were negatively related to subsequent test performance. It is possible that individual differences in need for achievement or attributional style account for discrepancies in the literature (see subsequent discussions of work by Dweck and colleagues).

Self-efficacy Literature

The relationship between attributions and academic performance also was examined in a series of studies by Schunk and colleagues. These studies focused on the impact of self-efficacy expectancies, defined by Bandura (1977, 1982) as expectations about one's ability to perform a certain task, on academic behavior in children. The majority of these studies (Bandura & Schunk, 1981; Schunk, 1981, 1982, 1983, 1984) assessed responses of children identified by their teachers as deficient in mathematical ability. Once identified, the children participated in instructional programs designed to improve their skills. They were asked prior to and following the training to estimate their ability to solve designated types of math problems. Although results varied somewhat, most of the work showed that self-efficacy expectancies provided by children at posttraining were signficant predictors of the children's accuracy at solving test problems provided after training (Schunk, 1981, 1982, 1983). Of particular interest was the finding in one study that self-efficacy expectancies were better predictors of children's problem-solving accuracy than their actual performance during the instructional sessions (Bandura & Schunk, 1981). Thus, despite what they had actually done during the training phases, children who had stronger expectancies about their ability to do the math problems were more likely to perform better on test problems administered following training.

These studies suggested that expectations about ability, sometimes regardless of actual performance outcome, had a significant impact on future academic performance. By definition, self-efficacy expectancies should be equivalent to attributions for ability, and in fact most measures of self-efficacy expectancies involved questions such as "How much do you believe you are capable of doing behavior X?" However, Schunk (1983) suggested that such expectancies may involve a conglomeration of attributions, the sum of which is what one thinks he/she can do given the status of perceived causes such as ability, effort, luck, and task difficulty. Such an hypothesis makes intuitive sense since in our own lives we know that merely by saying, "Yes, I can do behavior X," we do not mean necessarily that we are excessively confident in our ability to do behavior X. Rather, the behavior of which we are speaking may be perceived as an easy task that will require little effort or ability on our part. On the other hand, the statement, "I can do behavior X" also implies that one has *some* ability, regardless of the status of other causes. In fact, Schunk's work supported the centrality of attributions to ability as impacting on self-efficacy expectancies. Training children to attribute their math performance to effort did not consistently lead to increases in self-efficacy judgments (e.g., Schunk, 1981) (although in Schunk, 1982, training children in such a way did have some impact on self-efficacy statements). In addition, when training included teaching children to attribute their math performance to ability, self-efficacy expectancies were enhanced (e.g., Schunk, 1983, 1984).

Although the self-efficacy literature regarding children's achievement behavior sheds some light on the relationship between attributions and academic performance, the fact that self-efficacy expectancies probably involve additional attributional components muddies the water. In addition, all of the Schunk studies involved training children who already were identified as having deficient math skills. These children may have been particularly sensitive to ability-relevant information and may have reacted differently than children designated as nondeficient. The importance of individual differences such as these in understanding the relationship between attributions and academic performance is highlighted in the work of Dweck and colleagues, who examined the relationships from a learned-helplessness perspective.

Learned Helplessness and Individual Differences in Attributional Style

The phenomenon of learned helplessness and the role of attributions in the reformulated model of learned helplessness were reviewed in chapter 7 and will not be reiterated here. However, this model was applied to behavior in the achievement domain by Dweck and colleagues. In an early study, Dweck and Repucci (1973) administered a combination of solvable and unsolvable Wechsler Intelligence Scale for Children—Revised (WISC-R) block-design problems to a group of children. Initially, solvable and unsolvable problems were presented by separate experimenters (a "success experimenter" and a "failure experimenter"). When this pattern was broken, however, and the failure experimenter began to administer solvable problems, some children demonstrated an inability to solve the problems even though they were able to solve similar problems given by the success experimenter. These children demonstrated what appeared to be a helpless response. They were not actually less capable, but somehow perceived themselves to be so. Other children, on the other hand, had no difficulty completing accurately the solvable problems administered by the failure experimenter.

In an attempt to discover the reason for these differences in behavior, Dweck and Repucci (1973) divided the children into two groups based on their responses to the solvable problems given by the failure experimenter. These groups, characterized as either helpless or mastery-oriented, then were examined with regard to attributional styles. Results indicated that the mastery-oriented children in general took more responsibility for both success and failure whereas the helpless children were more likely to attribute their performance to external causes not under their control. With respect to attributions to internal causes, the mastery-oriented children attributed both success and failure more to effort when compared to helpless children, again indicating that the latter group felt less personally responsible for their performance. The groups did not differ, however, with regard to attributions to ability for either success or failure outcomes.

In subsequent studies it was demonstrated that helpless and mastery-oriented children utilized equivalent problem-solving strategies if they were asked initially to solve solvable problems (Diener & Dweck, 1978, 1980). However, when the children were given subsequent experience with failure (i.e., asked to solve unsolvable problems), problem-solving strategies differed significantly between the two groups. Over time with repeated failure experiences, helpless children deteriorated in performance and demonstrated the use of more ineffectual strategies. Mastery-oriented children, however, did not show similar deterioration and in fact some showed the use of even more sophisticated problem-solving strategies (Diener & Dweck, 1978, 1980). When asked to make attributions for failure, 50% of the helpless children attributed such outcomes to lack of ability whereas none of the mastery-oriented children did the same. Rather, these children attributed failure to low effort, bad luck, or unfairness on the part of the experimenter (Diener & Dweck, 1978).

In a separate experiment (Diener & Dweck, 1978) children were asked to "think aloud" as they attempted to solve the unsolvable problems. Significant differences in the nature of self-statements were observed between the two groups. Helpless children were more likely to verbalize attributional statements and two-thirds of them verbalized some kind of negative affect. Mastery-oriented children, however, did not make any attributional statements. Rather, the majority of these children verbalized statements of self-instruction and self-monitoring, apparently attempting to remedy rather than explain their failure.

When the children were asked to evaluate their initial success experiences, group differences also were apparent. Helpless children believed that other children would do better than themselves on similar problems, whereas mastery children perceived that other children would perform more poorly than themselves. Mastery children also had higher expectations for their own future performance than helpless children and demonstrated more accuracy in judging the number of problems they had solved correctly. Helpless children, however, underestimated the number of successes they had experienced and overestimated the number of failures.

Other groups of researchers provided data complementing the work from Dweck and colleagues. For example, Frieze and Snyder (1980) reported that high-ability children (designated as such on the basis of IQ scores) were more likely to take personal responsibility (make internal attributions) for success than failure, although such a pattern did not occur in low-ability children. Fielstein et al. (1985) reported that children characterized as having high self-esteem attributed academic success more to ability than did children identified as having low esteem. Conversely, the latter group was more likely to attribute such success to good luck.

Origins of Individual Differences

The data reviewed so far provided support for the notion that individual differences in attributional styles exist among children and that these styles are related significantly to performance of the children on academic tasks. The next question to be addressed involves the origins of variations in attributional style. Dweck and colleagues (e.g., Dweck & Bush, 1976; Dweck, Davidson, Nelson, & Enna, 1978) examined this question by evaluating differences in the nature and possible origin of gender-related attributional styles. Data from a number of studies suggested that female children were more likely to exhibit a helpless style of performance and attribution than males (Dweck & Repucci, 1973; Frey & Ruble, 1987; Power & Wagner, 1984). Dweck and Bush (1976), however, reported that this pattern occurred only when evaluations of performance were provided by adults. When evaluators of performance were peers, male children demonstrated the helpless pattern of behavior. Thus, the attributional differences did not appear to result from generalized gender-related traits. Rather, there appeared to be something about the nature of adult evaluations of female children that was associated with the helpless pattern exhibited by them.

Dweck et al. (1978) conducted two experiments to examine the nature of adult evaluations of both male and female children. First, in an observational experiment they found that teachers provided the same amount of absolute feedback to children of both genders. However, boys received more negative feedback that was provided in an ambiguous, diffuse manner and more often was directed to conduct problems rather than to intellectual aspects of work. On the other hand, girls received very little negative feedback for conduct problems. The majority of their negative feedback instead was directed toward intellectual aspects of their work.

Other gender differences were apparent in the attributions made by teachers for intellectual failure. For boys failure was attributed to inadequate effort eight times more often than for girls. In addition, approximately 55% of work-related criticism provided to boys made reference to intellectual inadequacy whereas 89% of work-related criticism given girls referred to the same. Hence, it appeared that boys were given more diffuse negative feedback that was directed at inadequate ability significantly less often than the negative feedback provided to girls. It may have been that boys learned to attribute negative feedback more to the teacher's general attitude toward them rather than to their own deficient skills. Girls, on the other hand, received very little negative feedback from teachers that was not directed specifically at their deficient ability and thus were more likely to attribute negative teacher evaluations to skill deficits.

In a second experiment, the authors tested the causal relationships suggested by these results (Dweck et al., 1978). Experimenters in a laboratory were programmed to exhibit a style of behavior similar to that observed in the prior experiment to be characteristic of teachers responding to either boys or girls. Both boys and girls then worked with an experimenter exhibiting either a "teacher-boy" or "teacher-girl" style. Results indicated that 75% of the children (regardless of gender) in the teacher-boy condition did not view their failure as being a result of deficient ability, and most often attributed failure to low effort. In the teacher-girl condition, 75% of the children attributed their failure to deficient ability, providing support for the notion that differential response styles on the part of adults might be responsible for gender-related patterns of attributions for academic performance.

A further study (Dweck, Goetz, & Strauss, 1980) addressed the question of transfer of attributions for failure from one situation to another. Results of this study indicated that following failure, girls recovered higher expectancies for success only when a new task was introduced, whereas boys recovered high expectancies for success either if a new task was introduced or if the evaluator of a familiar task was changed. These data suggested again that boys were unlikely to attribute failure to personal inability since they regained confidence in their ability to succeed when a new evaluator was introduced. Girls, however, were able to generate expectancies for success only if a new task was introduced, indicating their reliance on ability as an explanation for failure.

In a recent review, Dweck and Leggett (1988) described data demonstrating that the types of goals children pursue also determine whether they exhibit a helpless or mastery-oriented style of behavior and attributions. For instance, performance goals (in which children focused on attaining positive evaluations of their competence) coupled with perceptions of low ability produced the helpless pattern. On the other hand, learning goals (in which children focused on increasing their competence) led to the mastery-oriented pattern. Dweck and Leggett (1988) noted that performance goals also could produce a mastery style if ability levels were perceived to be adequate, although high confidence in ability might be difficult to maintain when one has a performance orientation.

Further, Dweck and Leggett (1988) described a model explaining the mechanisms through which differential goals lead to either helpless or mastery-oriented patterns. One aspect of this model of particular interest here suggested that goals are associated with attributional frameworks through which information is interpreted. For instance, Leggett and Dweck (1986) demonstrated that children with performance goals perceived an inverse relationship between effort and ability (exerting high effort means that one has little ability), whereas children with learning goals perceived a positive relationship between these two (exerting a lot of effort is a way to improve competence and ability). These goals seem to arise from differential theories regarding the fixed nature of intelligence—

that is, children with performance goals tend to view intelligence (and ability) as a fixed, unmodifiable entity, whereas children with learning goals perceive ability to be malleable and controllable (Bandura & Dweck, 1985).

These differential interpretive styles certainly would be expected to promote different behavioral patterns in response to challenging tasks. The performance goal pattern is likely to promote a helpless behavioral style given that failure on challenging tasks implies low ability that is uncontrollable, while learning goals create mastery-oriented behavior designed to increase levels of ability.

Concluding Points

The data to date suggest strongly that patterns of attribution have a significant impact on academic performance, and that attributional patterns may comprise personality variables that influence general academic ahievement. It also appears that patterns of adult behavior and type of achievement goals (performance vs. learning) can influence individual differences in attributional style. In the next section, we will review literature suggesting that these data can be effective in developing attribution-retraining programs designed to modify academic behavior.

Changing Attributions to Change Academic Behavior

In chapter 8, a number of experiments were reviewed that addressed the utility of various forms of attribution retraining to treat psychological difficulties. In this section, we will review similar studies that have attempted to retrain students with regard to attributional patterns for achievement behavior.

Given that helpless children give up in the face of failure, apparently because they attribute negative outcomes to ability deficits rather than to deficient effort (Diener & Dweck, 1978; Dweck & Repucci, 1973), it would seem useful to train these children to attribute academic failure to insufficient effort in an attempt to improve subsequent performance. Dweck (1975) conducted an experiment to test this idea. Twelve children, characterized as helpless by their school psychologist, principal, and classroom teacher, were divided into two groups and given one of two intensive training procedures.

Once identified as such, all helpless children were given 25 sessions of training which consisted either of repeated experience with success on math problems (designed to increase expectancies for success and to decrease the aversive aspects of task performance associated with failure) or mixed experience with both success and failure, with failure always attributed by the experimenter to insufficient effort. After training was completed, only children who had received attribution retraining demonstrated a decrease in the amount of deterioration in performance following experience with failure. On the other hand, children who had been given repeated experience with success continued to show levels of deterioration in performance following failure that were equivalent to those exhibited at pretreatment. These data suggested that a training program designed to increase the frequency with which helpless children attribute failure to effort can improve their postfailure academic performance.

These findings were extended to college students in a study by Wilson and Linville (1982). In a single "treatment session," a group of college freshmen was told that academic difficulties during the freshman year were due to unstable causes (although no specific causes were delineated) and that academic performance typically improved throughout additional years of college. Information was provided through written communications as well as via videotapes of advanced students who described improvements in their own academic performance since freshman year. Results indicated that students exposed to this information performed better on sample Graduate Record Examination (GRE) questions administered subsequent to the training session than students who had no access to similar information. In addition, longer-term results indicated that "treated" subjects had higher grade-point averages at the end of the semester as well as at the end of two subsequent semesters than "untreated" subjects, and that the former students were less likely to drop out of college at the end of their second year than the latter group.

Using a similar single-session attribution training procedure, Noel, Forsyth, and Kelley (1987) instructed failing college students (who had received grades of "D" or "F" on the first two exams in a semester-long course) that poor performance was due to unstable, internal causes such as deficient effort and poor study habits, as well as insufficient self-motivation and help-seeking. Subjects who received this information obtained improved grades on subsequent course examinations compared to control students who were not provided with such information.

In two replications of their original study (designed to address methodological critiques of their work by Block and Lanning, 1984), Wilson and Linville (1985) found that the effects of a single session of attribution intervention upon drop-out rates were considerably weaker than originally believed. However, when covariance analyses were conducted to control for any differences in baseline grade-point averages, students exposed to the single session of attribution training demonstrated higher grades at the end of the semester than did students in a control group. In addition, effects of the treatment on performance of sample GRE problems were replicated.

An interesting additional point was evident, however, when sex differences were analyzed. These analyses revealed that males responded more strongly to the attribution training than females. Specifically, only males exhibited improved performance on sample GRE problems following training, and they also showed more improvement in grade-point average following treatment than females. These data can be interpreted as being in line with findings from Dweck and colleagues. If females are more apt to attribute failure to ability deficits, a single session of training designed to increase attributions of failure to insufficient effort may be a relatively weak intervention. On the other hand, if males are more apt to attribute failure to nonability causes, a single session of training which supports their beliefs may create a stronger effect. Females also may have less modifiable beliefs about various aspects of academic behavior. Some support for this contention was provided in Wilson and Linville's (1985) observation that females were less likely to be influenced by the treatment manipulation. In fact, the information presented to treatment subjects did not significantly change females' estimates of the percentage of college students who improve their grades over time. Males, on the other hand, did change their beliefs significantly to be more in line with information provided by the experimenter (i.e., following treatment, they endorsed more strongly the belief that college grades would improve over time). Hence, females seemed to hold fairly solid beliefs regarding grade improvement, whereas males were more easily influenced by information provided by the experimenters. If indeed these solidly held beliefs involve attribution of failure most strongly to skills deficits, these data suggest that attribution-retraining programs will have to take into account gender differences in order to maximize their efficacy.

Concluding Points

The data reviewed here focused largely on reattribution-training programs designed to modify attributions for failure. Other studies attempted to improve academic performance by revising attributions for success. Studies conducted with a self-efficacy paradigm suggested that both self-efficacy expectancies and math performance improved when successful outcomes were attributed to ability rather than to either effort or a combination of ability and effort (Schunk, 1983). One study also supported the efficacy of training children to attribute success to adequate effort (Schunk, 1982), but no manipulation checks were included to ensure that students had made the desired types of attributions. Miller, Brickman, and Bolen (1975) also provided evidence in favor of attribution-retraining treatment that incorporated instructions about attributions for success. These authors found that repeatedly attributing success either to ability or the motivation to do well resulted in significantly greater increases in self-esteem and test scores in second graders. Furthermore, training students to attribute success to ability was more effective in improving performance than instructing them to attribute success to effort.

In summary, a reasonable amount of data have indicated that attribution treatment interventions have some promise in terms of improving the academic potential performance of students. These programs need to incorporate training for the attribution of both success and failure, and need to take into account individual differences in attributional style.

General Summary

Data reviewed in this chapter suggested that attributions following academic performance can have a meaningful impact on expectancies for future performance, affective reactions, and subsequent achievement-related behavior. The majority of recent data suggests that these relationships are moderated by the dimensional aspects of attributions. Also, individual differences in achievement motivation and attributional style seem to have an impact on academic success and/or failure. We also have adequate data to suggest that maladaptive patterns of attributions can be modified via attributional-retraining programs.

Future research in this area seems to be moving in the direction of applying the relationships noted in the achievement domain to other areas of functioning. For example, Weiner (1986) discussed the applicability of his attributional theory of achievement motivation and emotion to areas such as parole decisions, depression, victimization, and cigarette smoking. (Attributions within a number of these areas are discussed in other chapters of this text.) In addition, Dweck and Leggett (1988) discussed the utility of their attributional–individual-difference model in examining children's responses within the social as well as the achievement domain.

A second thrust of future work in the attribution–achievement literature likely will concern additional investigations regarding the origin of certain attributional patterns. For example, Graham (1984) examined the impact of others' affective cues on the attributions made by children following their academic failure. She found that sympathy communicated by others induced attributions of failure to low ability whereas anger communicated by others led to attributions of failure to lack of effort. Weiner (1986) also has noted that further work needs to elucidate the role of affect in attributional responses and subsequent behavior.

In general, enough data has been collected to validate the importance of attributions within the achievement context. However, as was noted throughout the text, the data are not all consistent and certain questions remain regarding the impact of attributions on expectancies, affect, and behavior, the role played by individual differences, and the origins of differential attributional patterns. In addition, the generalizability of data to other areas of functioning also requires future investigation.

Part III The Future

10
Further Directions and Unresolved Questions

As we write this final chapter, the year is 1988. Sadly, it is the year of the death of Fritz Heider, founder of attribution theory. He was 91. As Edward Jones (1987) said in a retrospective review of Heider's (1958) *The Psychology of Interpersonal Relations*, it is incomprehensible to imagine what the field of social psychology would be like today were it not for this classic, enduring contribution. Would there even be an attribution theory? Jones and Davis's (1965) and Kelley's (1967) statements are classic works in their own right. Yet, each of these crucial 1960s statements principally was built on and was designed to elucidate and enhance the research possibilities of Heider's seminal ideas. Jones (1987) went on to observe that "features of attribution reasoning . . . are woven indelibly into the fabric of contemporary psychology" (p. 215).

We trust that the reader of this book will have a better sense of that indelible influence after examining the various contents of this book. To write about attribution in 1988 and to continue to do so well into the next century—as we will argue shall occur—represent a testament to Heider's inestimable contribution. As noted in chapter 2, the enduring importance of attribution theory is emphasized in Kelley's (1978) observation that an attributional type of analysis ". . . came out of phenomena that psychologists have looked at and tried to interpret. I just can't imagine that the phenomena that are hooked into that kind of cognition will change of be modified. They'll never go away . . . ." (p. 384). We agree with Kelley and believe in general that both the spectrum of phenomena hooked into attributional cognition and the nature of the cognition itself will become better understood as we approach the 21st century.

In this final chapter, we will mention some of the specific directions attribution theory and research may take into the 21st century and in so doing note some of the continuing unresolved questions. There are two overall types of further developments that almost certainly will continue to unfold in the next decade. First, as evidenced by some of the recent work we have reviewed, there is and likely will remain interest in basic process questions. Second, as we have discussed at some length in this book, it would appear that attribution ideas will continue to influence work on a variety of more applied questions.

Further Directions: Basic Theoretical Issues

One fertile direction that is being pursued vigorously, especially by British and European attribution theorists, concerns attribution is group and societal circumstances. This direction (what we will call the "British school" approach) is well-illustrated by the writings and edited works of Antaki (1981), Hewstone (1983, in press), and Jaspars, Fincham, and Hewstone (1983). Hewstone (in press) argues that attribution at all levels, including the intrapersonal, is social in nature. He suggests that attribution may be based on social information, that it is social because it usually is common to members of particular groups and societies, and that it is social in its reference or object (i.e., attribution usually is about people). This line of reasoning is cogent to us, although we are not sure many attribution theorists ever would seriously argue the opposite position—that is, that in some sense attribution is not a social phenomenon. Nonetheless, given the vast expanse of possibility for differences in attributional activity across dyads, small groups, large groups, and cultures, the direction articulated well by Hewstone deserves greater attention from North American scholars.

The British school approach is complemented quite well by the work of sociologically oriented attribution theorists (e.g., Crittenden, 1983; Stryker & Gottlieb, 1981), who have called attention to the conceptual relationship between attribution and symbolic-interactionism processes as analyzed by the early theorist G.H. Mead (1934). A basic tenet of symbolic interactionism is that meanings ascribed to an object reflect an interpretation of it in social circumstances and that people interpret events by means of the system of meanings they have acquired through social interaction (Crittenden, 1983). Similar to the thinking in the British school approach, the symbolic-interactional approach sees attribution as an intrinsically social activity in which meaning gets established or negotiated in interaction. On a less conceptual dimension, as Crittenden (1983) suggests, the attribution area continues to provide one of the sturdiest bridges for timely dialogue between sociological and psychological social psychology.

Another related promising direction for attribution theory is to explore more thoroughly the role of self-identity in attributional activity (Weary & Arkin, 1981). It seems likely that people's most crucial attributional activity often is concerned with construction, maintenance, or modification of their personal identities. This process no doubt involves the continual attributional dilemma found in the search for truth or, "Who am I and what is my value as a human being?" One of the most intriguing arenas for this work on the link between attribution and identity concerns the interpersonal conditions under which people are stigmatized (Jones et al. 1984).

In this examination of how people construct meaning, it would be useful if more work were done on possible links between attribution theory and Kelly's (1955) psychology of personal constructs (Harvey, 1989). Kelly defined a personal construct as "a way in which some things are construed as being alike and yet different from others" (1955, p. 105). For example, a person may have a construct of Mary as "gentle" but also entertain a construct of her husband Tom as "nongentle" or "aggressive." This construing process, that is viewed as idiosyncratic to the individual by Kelly, bears some similarity to the attribution process proposed by Heider and others. However, in the history of these two major schools of thought in psychology, there has been little analysis of their relationship.

As reviews by Ross and Fletcher (1985) and Olson and Ross (1985) have discussed in depth, there always will be unresolved questions facing the classic theories of attribution. By design these theories are oversimplified conceptions of complex phenomena. Hence, it is likely that work will continue to refine those theories and their central elements. Below is a brief list of directions that we believe deserve more scrutiny by attribution scholars in coming years:

1. Integration of more molar and more molecular approaches to attribution (i.e., linking traditional positions with more recent theorizing that emphasizes social cognition in a fairly narrow sense). This relates to our discussion in chapter 3.
2. Incorporation of attribution-processes ideas into more general conceptions of cognitive processes, and in so doing better articulate how possible cognitive limitations affect attribution processes (also discussed in part in chapter 3).
3. Analysis of and research on dimensions of causality (complexity and multidimensionality of causal explanations as well as domain-specificity issues).
4. Work on attribution and individual differences and styles represents a potentially fertile direction, as suggested in chapter 7. Evidence derived from use of the Attribution Style Questionnaire has implicated a spectrum of possible individual-difference phenomena, although this work has not gone without challenge (e.g., Curtona et al., 1985). Another individual-style scale that would seem to have much potential has been developed by Fletcher et al. (1986). They demonstrated that people may differ in the degree of complexity with which they make attributions.
5. Interpersonal consequences of attributions (e.g., the interesting work on "attributional chains" done by Brickman, Ryan, & Wortman, 1975; Vinokur & Ajzen, 1982).
6. As discussed in chapter 4, further work is needed on the relationships among perceived causation, perceived responsibility, and blame assignment as developmental phenomena and in complex social settings.

Related to work on interpersonal consequences of attribution, the topic of accounts in close relationships represents yet another promising area for theoretical advance, as well as providing a naturalistic type of measurement technique. Theoretically, do accounts as "packages of attributions and other material" involve similar psychological processes that have been pinpointed in work on more isolated attributional responses? In addition to the work on accounts in relationships, several other lines of work on people's accounts have been pursued in the 1980s. For example, Felson and Ribner (1981) have studied prison inmates' explanations for their violent behavior. Lau and Russell (1980) studied excuses and justifications offered by athletes and reported in the sports pages of newspapers. More generally, Semin and Manstead (1984) have discussed accounts in a theory of accountability of conduct, and Gergen (1988) has discussed the overall merit of the case for analysis of narrative explanation in attribution theory. We believe that as more naturalistic settings and events are examined by attribution scholars, they will find that people do not simply attribute causes and responsibility; they also offer more elaborate accounts and stories. Eventually, research on more elaborate attributional responses may be used to help provide evidence about causal structures (e.g., for a discussion of such structures, see Antaki, 1986; Green, Lightfoot, Bandy, & Buchanan, 1985; Kelley, 1983). Free-response measures may facilitate probing of people's use of certain patterns of logic in making attributions (or, possibly more apropos, patterns of "psycho-logic," to use Abelson & Rosenberg's, 1958, term that was created to describe principles of cognitive consistency that exist in attitudinal–cognitive structures). These types of methods may permit more comprehensive and representative data regarding causal structure to be obtained. Whether examined by free-response methods or more structured methods, these causal structures represent an intriguing topic deserving greater attention among attribution theorists.

Probably the most intriguing avenue for past research on basic attributional problems has concerned bias in the attributional process. As was detailed in chapter 2, issues such as the role of cognitive and motivational factors in the operation of attributional biases have led to vigorous programs of research. This work likely will continue, and it may continue to point to the numerous areas in which people do not use formal kinds of attributional processes (Fiske & Taylor, 1984; Taylor, 1981). This line of work also is important because, as noted in chapter 2, we are learning much from it about the possible value of illusion in attributional processes. Apparently, we need our illusions almost as much as we need our realities in interpretive activity. A last issue with regard to bias, Quattrone (1982) has argued persuasively for the study of behavioral consequences of attributional biases. We heartily endorse his reasoning.

Finally, Harvey and Weary (1984) argued that at that point in time, there was a great need for work on attribution and behavior relationships.

In recent years, we have seen the development of some fine and relevant methodological approaches (e.g., see Ickes, in press, for a description of one of the most sophisticated approaches presently available for measurement both of behavior and cognitive–emotional variables, including attributions, in laboratory settings). Nonetheless, the attribution–behavior relationship still has not received the attention it deserves. It is a difficult chore to do causal investigations of this relationship via laboratory or field research. But such a step is necessary in this area, even as it was for the attitudes–behavior question.

Further Directions: Applications

In this volume, our coverage of the many new applications of attributional ideas has summarized only part of the recent developments. In the chapters on attribution and health-reflated functioning and attribution and close relationships, we have noted many new, fertile directions for the applications of attributional ideas and basic research. For example, there still is needed much work on the causal-direction question between attributions and related health behaviors. As mentioned in chapter 6, if attributions are causes of health developments (and the evidence thus far is not conclusive), it follows that therapeutic interventions at the attributional level may be effective. Furthermore, in addition to the work discussed in the chapters on the development of disfunctioning and treatment, there continues to be considerable dialogue regarding the potential utility and merit of attributional concepts in clinical psychology in general (e.g., Försterling, 1985, 1986; Harvey & Galvin, 1984).

At this point, we should emphasize that there are several additional strands of work on applications that have not been described. A few will be mentioned here. One such strand that has promise is Blank's (1987) application of attributional reasoning to a theory of life-span social psychology. In his analysis, he discusses possibly different attributional patterns about persons of different ages. For example, we have little available evidence on attributions made by persons of different ages, including the elderly, and/or about targets who vary in age. Would well-known patterns such as the actor–observer effect be replicated with individuals at later stages of life? As Blank points out, in this aging society we particularly need research to examine attributional processes in older persons.

Another type of application not discussed in this book concerns attribution's role in industrial settings involving management–worker interaction and relations and in organizational settings in general. For instance, do supervisor's attributions about subordinates' performances affect in direct ways the supervisors' subsequent behavior toward the subordinates? Intuition says "yes," and such questions increasingly have been asked by scholars in introducing attributional-type concepts into writings and research on organizational psychology (e.g., Deci, 1975; Heerwagen, Beach, & Mitchell, 1985). However, thus far the effort has not been related well to more mainstream attributional theory and research. Simply, one useful, consolidating step would be publication of an integrative *Psychological-Bulletin*-type review of this literature.

How do attributions interact with environmental influences to affect behavior? As environmental psychologists increasingly have emphasized multifaceted responses to environmental conditions, cognitive-attributional activity has begun to take on a prominent role in theorizing. For example, such activity may facilitate an enhancement of mood and behavioral functioning in the face of environmental stressors (Baum, Gatchel, Aiello, & Thompson, 1981; Ittleson, Proshansky, Rivlin, & Winkel, 1974; Lazarus, 1966).

Finally, an interesting strand of recent work has revealed how self-perception/attribution-type manipulations may be used to alleviate social anxiety in college-age men (Montgomery & Haemmerlie, 1986). Essentially, this approach has involved inducing men to make attributions of efficacy to their newly learned patterns of dating-approach behavior (see our related discussion of attributions and achievement in chapter 9).

Indeed, in the arena of applications of psychological knowledge, there has been a virtual smorgasbord of phenomena that have been treated with attribution-type concepts and reasoning in the last 2 decades. Some of these applications seem no more specific to attribution than to any general cognitive construct, while some others are highly specific to the contents of the attributional analyses developed by Heider, Jones, Kelley, Bem, Weiner, and other pioneers in the area. In principle, we see no problem with these many applications that, as noted in chapter 1, refer more to "attributional" theories than they do to "attribution" theory in its classic form.

Final Thoughts

It should be obvious to the reader by this time that there are many further directions and unresolved issues for attribution scholars. The attribution approach, as we have argued from chapter 1, is not that of a monolithic theory. Rather, it represents several general conceptions and a vast literature of research that together provide an exceedingly useful set of ideas for understanding how people think about and understand events, big and small, personal and social. We believe that this approach's flexibility and generality are positive features because they permit such a range of inter-relationships to be conceived. For example, the attribution approach may be related usefully to Kelly's (1955) personal-construct psychology; Klinger's (1977) and Frankl's (1963) "search for meaning" theses; Seligman and colleagues' learned helplessness; Schachter's (1964) theory of emotion; Bandura's (1986) self-efficacy theory; Mead's (1934) symbolic interactionism; and so on. In the end, the beauty of attribution theory and research is that of breadth and useful interconnectedness to much of the body of psychological knowledge that emphasizes the human mind and its operations. In all of psychological literature, the attributional approach also most centrally speaks to the facts of people's continual interpretation and assignment of meaning to their life situations and enduring ascriptions to self and others. We strongly believe that such qualities will continue to make the attribution approach a vital part of social psychological inquiry well into the next century.

References

Abelson, R.P. (1976). Script processing in attitude formation and decision-making. In J.S. Carroll & J.W. Payne (Eds.), *Cognition and social behavior* (pp. 33–46). Hillsdale, NJ: Erlbaum Associates.

Abelson, R.P., & Rosenberg, M.J. (1958). Symbolic psycho-logic: A model of attitudinal cognition. *Behavioral Science, 3*, 1–13.

Abramson, L.Y., & Sackheim, H.A. (1977). A paradox in depression: Uncontrollability and self-blame. *Psychological Bulletin, 84*, 835–851.

Abramson, L.Y., Seligman, M.E.P., & Teasdale, J.D. (1978). Learned helplessness in humans: Critique and reformulation. *Journal of Abnormal Psychology, 87*, 49–74.

Affleck, G., Allen, D. McGrade, B.J., & McQueeney, M. (1982). Maternal causal attributions at hospital discharge of high-risk infants. *American Journal of Mental Dificiency, 86*, 575–580.

Affleck, G., Allen, D.G., Tennen, H., McGrade, B.J., & Ratzan, S. (1985). Causal and control cognitions in parents' coping with chronically ill children. *Journal of Social and Clinical Psychology, 2*, 367–377.

Affleck, G., Tennen, H., & Gershman, K. (1985). Cognitive adaptations to high-risk infants: The search for mastery, meaning, and protection from future harm. *American Journal of Mental Deficiency, 87*, 653–656.

Ajzen, I., & Holmes, W.H. (1976). Uniqueness of behavioral effects in causal attribution. *Journal of Personality, 44*, 98–108.

Allen, D.A., Tennen, H., McGrade, B.J., Affleck, G., & Ratzan, S. (1983). Parent and child perceptions of the management of juvenile diabetes. *Journal of Pediatric Psychology, 8*, 129–141.

Alloy, L.B., & Tabachnik, N. (1984). Assessment of covariation by humans and animals: The joint influence of prior expectations and current situational information. *Psychological Review, 91*, 112–149.

Altmaier, E.M., Leary, M.R., Forsyth, D.R., & Ansel, J.C. (1979). Attribution therapy: Effects of locus of control and timing of treatment. *Journal of counseling Psychology, 26*, 481–486.

Anderson, C.A. (1983a). The causal structure of situations: The generation of plausible causal attributions as a function of type of event situation. *Journal of Experimental Social Psychology, 19*, 185–203.

Anderson, C.A. (1983b). Motivational and performance deficits in interpersonal settings: The effects of attributional style. *Journal of Personality and Social Psychology, 45*, 1136–1147.

Anderson, C.A., & Arnoult, L.H. (1985). Attributional models of depression, loneliness, and shyness. In J.H. Harvey, & G. Weary (Eds.), *Attribution: Basic issues and applications* (pp. 235–280). Orlando, FL: Academic Press.

Anderson, C.A., Horowitz, L., & French, R. (1983). Attributional style of lonely and depressed people. *Journal of Personality and Social Psychology*, *45*, 127–136.

Anderson, C.A., Jennings, D.L., & Arnoult, L.H. (1988). The validity and utility of the attributional style construct at a moderate level of specificity. *Journal of Personality and Social Psychology*, *55*, 979–990.

Andreasen, N.J.C., Noyes, R., & Hartford, C.E. (1972). Factors influencing adjustment of burn patients during hospitalization. *Psychosomatic Medicine*, *43*, 517–525.

Antaki, C. (Ed.). (1981). *The psychology of ordinary explanations*. London: Academic Press.

Antaki, C. (1986). Ordinary explanation in conversation: Causal structures and their defence. *European Journal of Social Psychology*, *15*, 214–230.

Antaki, C. (1987). Types of accounts within relationships. In R. Burnett, D. Clark, & P. McGhee (Eds.), *Accounting for relationships* (pp. 97–133). London: Methuen.

Arkin, R.M., Appleman, A.J., & Burger, J.M. (1980). Social anxiety, self-presentation, and the self-serving bias in causal attributions. *Journal of Personality and Social Psychology*, *38*, 23–35.

Arkin, R.M., & Baumgardner, A.H. (1985). Self-handicapping. In J.H. Harvey & G. Weary (Eds.), *Attribution: Basic issues and applications* (pp. 169–202). Orlando, FL: Academic Press.

Arkin, R.M., & Maruyama, G.M. (1979). Attribution, affect, and college exam performance. *Journal of Educational Psychology*, *71*, 85–93.

Armsby, R.E. (1971). A reexamination of the development of moral judgments in children. *Child Development*, *42*, 1241–1248.

Arnkoff, D.B., & Mahoney, M.J. (1979). The role of perceived control in psychotherapy. In L.C. Perlmutter & R.A. Monty (Eds.), *Choice and perceived control* (pp. 155–174). Hillsdale, NJ: Erlbaum Associates.

Atkinson, J.W. (1964). *An introduction to motivation*. Princeton, NJ: Van Nostrand.

Attneave, F. (1959). *Applications of information theory to psychology*. New York: Holt, Rinehart, & Winston.

Averill, J.A. (1982). *Anger and aggression*. New York: Springer-Verlag.

Averill, J.A. (1983). Studies on anger and aggression. *American Psychologist*, *38*, 1145–1160.

Bailey, R.S., Helm, B., & Gladstone, R. (1975). The effects of success and failure in a real-life setting: Performance, attribution, affect, and expectancy. *Journal of Personality*, *89*, 137–147.

Baldwin, C.P., & Baldwin, A.L. (1970). Children's judgments of kindness. *Child Development*, *41*, 29–47.

Bandura, A. (1969). *Principles of behavior modification*. New York: Holt.

Bandura, A. (1977). Self-efficacy: Toward a unifying theory of behavior change. *Psychological Review*, *84*, 191–215.

Bandura, A. (1982). Self-efficacy mechanism in human agency. *American Psychologist*, *37*, 122–147.

Bandura, A. (1986). *Social foundations of thought and action: A social cognitive theory*. Englewood Cliffs, NJ: Prentice-Hall.

Bandura, A., & Dweck, C.S. (1985). *The relationship of conceptions of intelligence and achievement goals to achievement-related cognition, affect, and behavior.* Manuscript submitted for publication.

Bandura, A., Jeffrey, R.W., & Gajdos, E. (1975). Generalized change through participant modeling with self-directed mastery. *Behavior Research and Therapy, 13*, 141–152.

Bandura, A., & Schunk, D.H. (1981). Cultivating competence, self-efficacy, and intrinsic interest through proximal self-motivation. *Journal of Personality and Social Psychology, 41*, 586–598.

Barnett, P.A., & Gotlib, I.H. (1988). Psychosocial functioning and depression: Distinguishing among antecedents, concomitants, and consequences. *Psychological Bulletin, 104*, 97–126.

Baron, R.M. (1980). Contrasting approaches to social knowing: An ecological perspective. *Personality and Social Psychology Bulletin, 6*, 590–600.

Baum, A., Gatchel, R.J., Aiello, J.R., & Thompson, D. (1981). Cognitive mediation of environmental stress. In J.H. Harvey (Ed.), *Cognition, social behavior, and the environment* (pp. 513–534). Hillsdale, NJ: Erlbaum Associates.

Baumgardner, A.H., Heppner, P.P., & Arkin, R.M. (1986). Role of causal attribution in personal problem solving. *Journal of Personality and Social Psychology, 50*, 636–643.

Baumgardner, A.H., Lake, E.A., & Arkin, R.M. (1984). *Claiming depression as a self-handicap.* Unpublished manuscript, University of Missouri, Columbia.

Beach, S.R.H., Abramson, L.Y., & Levine, F.M. (1981). The attributional reformulation of learned helplessness: Therapeutic implications. In H. Glazer & J. Clarkin (Eds.), *Depression: Behavioral and directive intervention strategies* (pp. 131–166). New York: Garland Press.

Beck, A.T., & Beck, R.W. (1972). Screening depressed patients in family practice: A rapid technic. *Postgraduate Medicine, 52*, 81–85.

Beck, A.T., Rush, A.J., Shaw, B.F., & Emery, G. (1979). *Cognitive therapy of depression.* New York: Guilford Press.

Beery, R.G. (1975). Fear of failure in the student experience. *Personnel and Guidance Journal, 54*, 190–203.

Bem, D.J. (1967a). Reply to Judson Mills. *Psychological Review, 74*, 536–537.

Bem, D.J. (1967b). Self-perception: An alternative interpretation of cognitive dissonance phenomena. *Psychological Review, 74*, 183–200.

Bem, D.J. (1972). Self-perception theory. In L. Berkowitz (Ed.), *Advances in experimental social psychology (Vol. 6)* (pp. 1–62). New York: Academic Press.

Bem, D.J., & McConnell, H.K. (1970). On the salience of premanipulation attitudes. *Journal of Personality and Social Psychology, 14*, 23–31.

Benesh-Weiner, M. (Ed.). (1988). *Fritz Heider: The Notebook (Vols. 1–2).* New York: Springer-Verlag.

Berg-Cross, L.G. (1975). Intentionality, degree of damage, and moral judgments. *Child Development, 46*, 970–974.

Berglas, S. (1986). *The success syndrome: Hitting bottom when you reach the top.* New York: Plenum.

Berglas, S., & Jones, E.E. (1978). Drug choice as an internalization strategy in response to noncontingent success. *Journal of Personality and Social Psychology, 36*, 405–417.

Berley, R.A., & Jacobson, N.S. (1984). Causal attributions in intimate relationships: Toward a model of cognitive–behavioral marital therapy. In P.C. Kendall (Ed.), *Advances in cognitive–behavioral research and therapy (Vol. 3)* (pp. 1–60). Orlando, FL: Academic Press.

Bernstein, W.M., Stephan, W.G., & Davis, M.H. (1979). Explaining attributions for achievement: A path analytic approach. *Journal of Personality and Social Psychology, 37*, 1810–1821.

Berscheid, E., Graziano, W., Monson, T., & Dermer, M. (1976). Outcome dependency: Attention, attribution, and attraction. *Journal of Personality and Social Psychology, 34*, 978–989.

Blank, T.O. (1987). Attributions as dynamic elements in a lifespan social psychology. In R.P. Abeles (Ed.), *Life-span perspectives and social psychology* (pp. 61–84). Hillsdale, NJ: Erlbaum Associates.

Block, J., & Lanning, K. (1984). Attribution therapy requestioned: A secondary analysis of the Wilson–Linville study. *Journal of Personality and Social Psychology, 46*, 705–708.

Bootzin, R.R., Herman, C.P., & Nicassio, P. (1976). The power of suggestion: Another examination of misattribution and insomnia. *Journal of Personality and Social Psychology, 34*, 673–679.

Borgida, E., & Brekke, N. (1981). The base rate fallacy in attribution and prediction. In J.H. Harvey, W.J. Ickes, & R.F. Kidd (Eds.), *New directions in attribution research (Vol. 3)* (pp. 66–97). Hillsdale, NJ: Erlbaum Associates.

Bowers, K.S. (1979, August). Presenter in debate with Richard Nisbett *Introspective access to higher order cognitive processes: Do we tell more than we know?* Presented at the meeting of the American Psychological Association, New York.

Bradbury, T.N., & Fincham, F.D. (in press). Assessing spontaneous attributions in marital interaction: Methodological and conceptual considerations. *Journal of Social and Clinical Psychology, 7*, 122–130.

Braswell, L., Koehler, C., & Kendall, P.C. (1985). Attributions and outcomes in child psychotherapy. *Journal of Social and Clinical Psychology, 3*, 458–465.

Brehm, J.W. (1966). *A theory of psychological reactance.* New York: Academic Press.

Brehm, J.W. (1972). *Responses to loss of freedom: A theory of psychological reactance.* Morristown, NJ: General Learning Press.

Brehm, S.S. (1976). *The application of social psychology to clinical practice.* Washington: Hemisphere.

Brende, J.S., & Parson, E.R. (1985). *Vietnam veterans: The roads to recovery.* New York: Plenum.

Brendt, T.J., & Brendt, E.G. (1975). Children's use of motives and intentionality in person perception and moral judgment. *Child Development, 46*, 904–912.

Brewin, C.R. (1984). Attributions for industrial accidents: Their relationship to rehabilitation outcome. *Journal of Social and Clinical Psychology, 2*, 156–164.

Brewin C.R., & Antaki, C. (1987). An analysis of ordinary explanations in clinical attribution research. *Journal of Social and Clinical Psychology, 5*, 79–98.

Brickman, P.K., Ryan, K., & Wortman, C.B. (1975). Causal chains: Attributions of responsibility as a function of immediate and prior causes. *Journal of Personality and Social Psychology, 32*, 1060–1067.

Brodt, S.E., & Zimbardo, P.G. (1981). Modifying shyness-related social behavior through symptom misattribution. *Journal of Personality and Social Psychology, 41*, 437–449.

Bromfield, R., Weisz, J.R., & Messer, T. (1986). Children's judgments and attributions in response to the "mentally retarded" label: A developmental approach. *Journal of Abnormal Psychology*, *95*, 81–87.

Brown, J.D., & Seigel, J.M. (1988). Attributions for negative life events and depression: The role of perceived control. *Journal of Personality and Social Psychology*, *54*, 316–322.

Brown, J., & Weiner, B. (1984). Affective consequences of ability versus effort ascriptions: Controversies, resolutions, and quandaries. *Journal of Educational Psychology*, *76*, 146–158.

Brunson, B.I., & Matthews, K.A. (1981). The Type-A coronary-prone behavior pattern and reactions to uncontrollable stress: An analysis of performance strategies, affect, and attributions during failure. *Journal of Personality and Social Psychology*, *40*, 906–918.

Bugental, D.B. (1987). Attributions as moderator variables within social interactional systems. *Journal of Social and Clinical Psychology*, *5*, 469–484.

Burnett, R., McGhee, P., & Clarke, D.C. (Eds.). (1987). *Accounting for relationships*. London: Methuen.

Burns, D.B., & Beck A.T. (1978). Cognitive behavior modification of mood disorders. In J.P. Foreyt & D.P. Rathjen (Eds.), *Cognitive behavior therapy* (pp. 109–134). New York: Plenum Press.

Buss, A.R. (1978). Causes and reasons in attribution theory: A conceptual critique. *Journal of Personality and Social Psychology*, *36*, 1311–1321.

Calveric, B.R. (1979, September). *A developmental approach to conceptualizing others*. Paper presented at the American Psychological Association, New York, NY.

Calvert-Boyanowski, J., & Leventhal, H. (1975). The role of information in attenuating behavioral responses to stress: A reinterpretation of the misattribution phenomenon. *Journal of Personality and Social Psychology*, *32*, 69–75.

Cantor, J.R., Zillmann, D., & Bryant, J. (1975). Enhancement of experienced sexual arousal in response to erotic stimuli through misattribution of unrelated residual excitation. *Journal of Personality and Social Psychology*, *32*, 69–75.

Carver, C.S., DeGregorio, E., & Gillis, R. (1980). Field-study evidence of an ego-defensive bias in attribution among two categories of observers. *Personality and Social Psychology Bulletin*, *36*, 1311–1321.

Cate, B.M., Huston, T.L., & Nesselroade, J.R. (1986). Premarital relationships: Toward a typology of pathways to marriage. *Journal of Social and Clinical Psychology*, *4*, 3–22.

Chandler, M.J., Greenspan, M., & Barenboim, C. (1973). Judgments of intentionality in response to videotaped and verbally presented moral dilemmas: The medium is the message. *Child Development*, *44*, 315–320.

Christensen, A., Sullaway, M., & King, C. (1983). Systematic error in behavioral reports of dyadic interaction: Egocentric bias and content effects. *Behavioral Assessment*, *5*, 131–142.

Clark, M.S., & Reis, H.T. (1988). Interpersonal processes in close relationships. *Annual Review of Psychology*, *39*, 609–672.

Clary, E.G., & Tesser, A. (1983). Reactions to unexpected events: The naive scientist and interpretive activity. *Personality and Social Psychology Bulletin*, *9*, 609–620.

Cochran, S.D., & Hammen, C.L. (1985). Perceptions of stressful life events and depression: A test of attributional models. *Journal of Personality and Social Psychology*, *48*, 1562–1571.

Cohen, E.A., Gelfand, D.M., Hartmann, D.P., Partlow, M.E., Montemayor, R., & Shigetomi, C.C. (1977, March). *Children's causal reasoning.* Paper presented at the biennial meeting of the Society for Research in Child Development, San Francisco, CA.

Cohen, E.A., Gelfand, D.M., & Hartmann, D.P. (1979, September). *Developmental differences in children's causal attributions.* Paper presented at the meeting of the American Psychological Association, New York, NY.

Cohen, J.L., Dowling, N., Bishop, G., & Maney, W.J. (1985). Causal attributions: Effects of self-focused attentiveness and self-esteem feedback. *Personality and Social Psychology Bulletin*, *11*, 369–378.

Colletti, G., & Kopel, S.A. (1979). Maintaining behavior change: An investigation of three maintenance strategies and the relationship of self-attribution to the long-term reduction of cigarette smoking. *Journal of Experimental Social Psychology*, *47*, 614–617.

Condiotte, M.M., & Lichtenstein, E. (1981). Self-efficacy and relapse in smoking cessation programs. *Journal of Consulting and Clinical Psychology*, *49*, 648–658.

Conger, J.C., Conger, A.J., & Brehm, S. (1976). Fear level as a moderator of false feedback effects in snake phobics. *Journal of Consulting and Clinical Psychology*, *44*, 135–141.

Copple, C.E., & Coon, R.C. (1977). The role of causality in encoding and re-membering events as a function of age. *Journal of Genetic Psychology*, *130*, 129–136.

Costanzo, P., Coie, J., Grumet, S., & Farnill, D. (1973). A reexamination of the effects of intent and consequence on children's moral judgment. *Child Development*, *44*, 154–161.

Costanzo, P.R., & Dix, T.H. (1983). Beyond the information processed: Socialization in the development of attributional processes. In E. Tory Higgins, D.N. Ruble, & W.W. Hartup (Eds.), *Social cognition and social development: A sociocultural perspective* (pp. 63–81). Cambridge: Cambridge University Press.

Cotton, J.L. (1981). A review of research on Schachter's theory of emotion and the misattribution of arousal. *European Journal of Social Psychology*, *11*, 365–397.

Covington, M.V., & Beery, R. (1976). *Self-worth and school learning.* New York: Holt, Reinhart, & Winston.

Covington, M.V., & Omelish, C.L. (1979a). Effort: The double-edged sword in school achievement. *Journal of Educational Psychology*, *71*, 169–182.

Covington, M.V., & Omelich, C.L. (1979b). It's best to be able and virtuous too: Student and teacher evaluative responses to successful effort. *Journal of Educational Psychology*, *71*, 688–700.

Covington, M.V., & Omelich, C.L. (1984). Controversies or consistencies? A reply to Brown and Weiner. *Journal of Educational Psychology*, *76*, 159–168.

Coyne, J.C., & Gotlib, I.H. (1983). The role of cognition in depression: A critical appraisal. *Psychological Bulletin*, *94*, 472–505.

Crittenden, K.S. (1983). Sociological aspects of attribution. *Annual Review of Sociology*, *9*, 425–446.

Crocker, J. (1981). Judgment of covariation by social perceivers. *Psychological Bulletin*, *90*, 272–292.

Croog, S.H., & Richards, N.P. (1977). Health beliefs and smoking patterns in heart patients and their wives: A longitudinal study. *American Journal of Public Health*, *67*, 921–930.

Cunningham, J.D., & Kelley, H.H. (1975). Causal attributions for interpersonal events of varying magnitudes. *Journal of Personality*, *43*, 74–93.

Cunningham, J.D., Starr, P.A., & Kanouse, D.E. (1979). Self as actor, active observer, and passive observer: Implications for causal attributions. *Journal of Personality and Social Psychology*, *37*, 1146–1159.

Cutrona, C.E., Russell, D., & Jones, R.D. (1985). Cross-situational consistency in causal attributions: Does attributional style exist? *Journal of Personality and Social Psychology*, *47*, 1043–1053.

Darley, J.M., & Latane, B. (1968). Bystander intervention in emergencies: Diffusion of responsibility. *Journal of Personality and Social Psychology*, *8*, 74–93.

Davies, J.B. (1982). Alcoholism, social policy, and intervention. In J.R. Eiser (Ed.), *Social psychology and behavioral medicine* (pp. 235–260). London: Wiley.

Davison, G., Tsujimoto, R.N., & Glaros, A.G. (1973). Attribution and the maintenance of behavior change in falling asleep. *Journal of Personality and Social Psychology*, *82*, 124–133.

Davison, G., & Valins, S. (1969). Maintenance of self-attributed and drug attributed behavior change. *Journal of Personality and Social Psychology*, *11*, 25–33.

Deaux, K. (1976). Sex: A perceptive on the attribution process. In J.H. Harvey, E.J. Ickes, & R.F. Kidd (Eds.), *New directions in attribution research (Vol. 1)* (pp. 335–352). Hillsdale, NJ: Erlbaum Associates.

Deaux, K., & Major, B. (1977). Sex-related patterns in the unit of perception. *Personality and Social Psychology Bulletin*, *3*, 297–300.

Deci, E.L. (1975). *Intrinsic motivation*. New York: Plenum.

DiClemente, C.C., Prochaska, J.O., & Gibertini, M. (1985). Self-efficacy and the stages of self-change of smoking. *Cognitive Therapy and Research*, *9*, 181–200.

Diener, C.I., & Dweck, C.S. (1978). An analysis of learned helplessness: Continuous changes in performance, strategy, and achievement cognitions following failure. *Journal of Personality and Social Psychology*, *36*, 457–464.

Diener, C.I., & Dweck, C.S. (1980). An analysis of learned helplessness: II. The processing of success. *Journal of Personality and Social Psychology*, *39*, 940–952.

DiVitto, B., & McArthur, L.Z. (1978). Developmental differences in the use of distinctiveness, consensus, and consistency information. *Developmental Psychology*, *14*, 474–482.

Dix, T.H., & Grusec, J.E. (1985). Parent attribution processes in the socialization of children. In I.E. Sigel (Ed.), *Parental belief systems: The psychological consequences for children* (pp. 201–233). Hillsdale, NJ: Erlbaum Associates.

Dix, T., & Herzberger, S. (1983). The role of logic and salience in the development of causal attribution. *Child Development*, *54*, 960–967.

Doherty, W.J. (1982). Attribution style and negative problem solving in marriage. *Family Relations*, *31*, 23–27.

Dweck, C.S. (1975). The role of expectations and attributions in the alleviation of learned helplessness. *Journal of Personality and Social Psychology*, *31*, 674–685.

Dweck, C.S., & Bush, E.S. (1976). Sex differences in learned helplessness: I. Differential debilitation with peer and adult evaluators. *Developmental Psychology*, *12*, 147–156.

Dweck, C.S., Davidson, W., Nelson, S., & Enna, B. (1978). Sex differences in learned helplessness: II. The contingencies of evaluative feedback in the classroom and III. An experimental analysis. *Developmental Psychology*, *14*, 268–276.

Dweck, C.S., Goetz, T.E., & Strauss, N.L. (1980). Sex differences in learned helplessness: IV. An experimental and naturalistic study of failure generalization and its mediators. *Journal of Personality and Social Psychology*, *38*, 441–452.

Dweck, C.S., & Leggett, E.L. (1988). A social–cognitive approach to motivation and personality. *Psychological Review*, *95*, 256–273.

Dweck, C.S., & Licht, B. (1980). Learned helplessness and intellectual achievement. In J. Garber & M.E.P. Seligman (Eds.), *Human helplessness* (pp. 197–221). New York: Academic Press.

Dweck, C.S., & Repucci, N.D. (1973). Learned helplessness and reinforcement responsibility in children. *Journal of Personality and Social Psychology*. *25*, 109–116.

Ebbesen, E.B., & Allen, R.B. (1979). Cognitive processes in implicit personality and trait inferences. *Journal of Personality and Social Psychology*, *37*, 471–488.

Eisen, S.V. (1979). Actor–observer difference in information inference and causal attribution. *Journal of Personality and Social Psychology*, *37*, 261–272.

Eiser, J.R., & van der Pligt, J. (1986). Smoking cessation and smokers' perceptions of their addiction. *Journal of Social and Clinical Psychology*, *4*, 60–70.

Eiser, J.R., van der Pligt, J., Raw, M., & Sutton, S.R. (1985). Trying to stop smoking: Effects of perceived addiction, attributions for failure, and expectancy of success. *Journal of Behavioral Medicine*, *8*, 321–341.

Elig, T. & Frieze, I. (1975). A multidimensional scheme for coding and interpreting perceived causality for success and failure events: The CSPS. *Catalogue of Selected Documents in Psychology*, *5*, 213.

Elig, T.W., & Frieze, I.H. (1979). Measuring causal attributions for success and failure. *Journal of Personality and Social Psychology*, *37*, 621–634.

Ellis, A. (1962). *Reason and emotion in psychotherapy*. New York: Lyle Stuart Press.

Enzle, M.E., Harvey, M.D., & Wright, E.F. (1980). Personalism and distinctiveness. *Journal of Personality and Social Psychology*, *39*, 542–552.

Eysenck, H.J. (1987). Anxiety, learned helplessness, and cancer: A causal theory. *Journal of Anxiety Disorders*, *1*, 87–104.

Farnill, D. (1974). The effects of social-judgment set on children's use of intent information. *Journal of Personality*, *42*, 276–289.

Felson, R.B., & Ribner, S.A. (1981). An attributional approach to accounts and sanctions for criminal violence. *Social Psychology Quarterly*, *44*, 137–142.

Fiedler, K. (1982). Causal schemata: Review and criticism of research on a popular construct. *Journal of Personality and Social Psychology*, *42*, 1001–1013.

Fielstein, E., Klein, M.S., Fischer, M., Hanan, C., Koburger, P., Schneider, M.J., & Leitenberg, H. (1985). Self-esteem and causal attributions for success and failure in children. *Cognitive Therapy and Research*, *9*, 381–398.

Fincham, F.D. (1981). Perception and moral evaluation in young children. *British Journal of Social Psychology*, *20*, 265–270.

Fincham, F.D. (1982b). Responsibility attribution in the culturally deprived. *The Journal of Genetic Psychology*, *140*, 229–235.

Fincham, F.D. (1982a). Moral judgment and the development of causal schemes. *European Journal of Social Psychology*, *12*, 47–61.

Fincham, F.D. (1983a). Developmental dimensions of attribution theory. In J. Jaspers, F. Fincham, & M. Hewstone (Eds.), *Attribution theory and research: Conceptual, Development, and social dimensions* (pp. 117–164). London: Academic Press.

Fincham, F.D. (1983b). Clinical applications of attribution theory: Problems and perspectives. In M. Hewstone (Ed.), *Attribution theory: Extensions and applications* (pp. 187–205). Oxford: Blackwells.

Fincham, F.D. (1985a). Outcome valence and situational constraints on the responsibility attributions of children and adults. *Social Cognition, 3,* 218–133.

Fincham, F.D. (1985b). Attributions in close relationships. In J.H. Harvey & G. Weary (Eds.), *Attribution: Basic issues and applications* (pp. 203–234). New York: Academic Press.

Fincham, F.D., & Beach, S.R. (in press). Attribution processes in distressed and nondistressed couples: Real versus hypothetical events. *Cognitive Therapy and Research.*

Fincham, F.D., Beach, S.R., & Baucom, D.H. (1987). Attribution processes in distressed and nondistressed couples: Self-partner attribution differences. *Journal of Personality and Social Psychology, 52,* 739–748.

Fincham, F.D., & Bradbury, T.N. (1987). The impact of attributions in marriage: A longitudinal analysis. *Journal of Personality and Social Psychology, 53,* 510–517.

Fincham, F.D., & Bradbury, T.N. (in press). Cognition in marriage: A program of research on attributions. In D. Perlman & W. Jones (Eds.), *Advances in personal relationships (Vol. 2).* Greenwich, CT: JAI Press.

Fincham, F.D., & Cain, K.M. (1986). Learned helplessness in humans: A developmental analysis. *Developmental Review, 6,* 301–333.

Fincham, F., & Jaspars, J. (1979). Attribution of responsibility to the self and other in children and adults. *Journal of Personality and Social Psychology, 37,* 1589–1602.

Fincham, F., & O'Leary, K.D., (1983). Causal inferences for spouse behavior in maritally distressed and nondistressed couples. *Journal of Social and Clinical Psychology, 1,* 32–57.

Fincham, F.D., & Roberts, C. (1985). Intervening causation and the mitigation of responsibility for harm doing. II. The role of limited mental capacities. *Journal of Experimental Social Psychology, 21,* 178–194.

Fincham, F.D., & Shultz, T.R. (1981). Intervening causation and the mitigation of responsibility for harm. *British Journal of Social Psychology, 20,* 113–120.

Firth, J. & Brewin, C. (1982). Attributions and recovery from depression: A preliminary study using cross-lagged correlationl analysis. *British Journal of Clinical Psychology, 21,* 229–230.

Fiske, S.T., Kenny, D.A., & Taylor, S.E. (1982). Structural models for the mediation of salience effects on attribution. *Journal of Experimental Social Psychology, 18,* 105–127.

Fiske, S.T., & Taylor, S.E. (1984). *Social cognition.* New York: Random House.

Fitzgerald, N.M., & Surra, C.A. (1981, November). *Studying the development of dyadic relationships.* Paper presented at the National Council on Family Relations, Milwaukee, WI.

Fletcher, G.J.O. (1983). The analysis of verbal explanations for marital separation: Implications for attribution theory. *Journal of Applied Social Psychology, 13,* 245–258.

Fletcher, G.J.O., Danilovics, P., Fernandez, G., Peterson, D., & Reeder, G.D. (1986). Attributional complexity: An individual differences measure. *Journal of Personality and Social Psychology, 51*, 875–884.

Fletcher, G.J.O., Fincham, F.D., Cramer, L., & Heron, W. (1987). The role of attributions in the development of dating relationships. *Journal of Personality and Social Psychology, 53*, 481–489.

Folkes, V.S. (1982). Communicating the reasons for social rejection. *Journal of Experimental Social Psychology, 18*, 235–252.

Forsterling, F. (1985). Attributional retraining: A review. *Psychological Bulletin, 98*, 495–512.

Forsterling, F. (1986). Attributional conceptions in clinical psychology. *American Psychologist, 41*, 275–285.

Forsyth, D.R. (1986). An attributional analysis of students' reactions to success and failure. In R.S. Feldman (Ed.), *Social Psychology of Education* (pp. 17–38). New York: Cambridge University Press.

Forsyth, D.R., Berger, R.E., & Mitchell, T. (1981). The effects of self-serving vs. Other-serving claims of responsibility on attraction and attribution in groups. *Social Psychology Quarterly, 44*, 59–64.

Forsyth, D.R., & McMillan, J.H. (1981a). Attributing affect and expectations: A test of Weiner's three-dimensional model. *Journal of Educational Psychology, 73*, 393–403.

Forsyth, D.R., & McMillan, J.H. (1981b). The attribution cube and reactions to educational outcomes. *Journal of Educational Psychology, 73*, 632–641.

Forsyth, D.R., & McMillan, J.H. (1982, August). *Reactions to educational outcomes: Some affective and attributional correlates.* Paper presented at the annual meeting of the American Psychological Association, Washington, D.C. [Cited in D.R. Forsyth (1986), An attributional analysis of students' reactions to success and failure. In R.S. Feldman (Ed.), *Social psychology of education.* New York: Cambridge University Press.]

Forsyth, N.L., & Forsyth, D.R. (1982). Internality, controllability and the effectiveness of attributional interpretations in counseling. *Journal of Counseling Psychology, 29*, 140–150.

Forsyth, N.L., & Forsyth, D.R. (1983). The promise and peril of attributional counseling: A reply. *Journal of Counseling Psychology, 30*, 457–458.

Frankl, V.E. (1963). *Man's search for meaning.* New York: Washington Square.

Frey, K.S., & Ruble, D.N. (1987). What children say about classroom performance: Sex and grade differences in perceived competence. *Child Development, 58*, 410–413.

Friedman, M., & Rosenman, R.H. (1974). *Type A behavior and your heart.* New York: Knopf.

Frieze, I. (1976). Causal attributions and information-seeking to explain success and failure. *Journal of Research in Personality, 10*, 293–305.

Frieze, I.H. (1979). Perceptions of battered wives. In I.H. Frieze, D. Bar-Tal, & J.S. Carroll (Eds.), *New approaches to social problems: Applications of attribution theory* (pp. 79–108). San Francisco: Jossey Bass.

Frieze, I.H., & Snyder, H.N. (1980). Children's beliefs about the causes of success and failure in school settings. *Journal of Educational Psychology, 72*, 186–196.

Frieze, I., & Weiner, B. (1971). Cue utilization and attributional judgments for success and failure. *Journal of Personality, 39*, 591–605.

Funder, D.C. (1982). On the accuracy of dispositional vs. situational attributions. *Social Cognition*, *1*, 205–222.

Funder, D.C. (1987). Errors and mistakes: Evaluating the accuracy of social judgment. *Psychological Bulletin*, *101*, 75–90.

Garber, J., Miller, W.R., & Seaman, S.F. (1979). Learned helplessness, stress, and the depressive disorders. In R.A. Depue (Ed.), *The psychobiology of the depressive disorders: Implications for the effects of stress* (pp. 335–364). New York: Academic Press.

Gaupp, L.A., Stern, R.M., & Galbraith, G.G. (1972). False heart-rate feedback and reciprocal inhibition by aversive relief in the treatment of snake avoidance behavior. *Behavior Therapy*, *3*, 7–20.

Gergen, M.M. (1988). Narrative structures in social explanation. In C. Antaki (Ed.), *Analysing everyday explanation* (pp. 94–112). London: Sage.

Gilbert, D.T., Jones, E.E., & Pelham, B.W. (1987). Influence and inference: What the active perceiver overlooks. *Journal of Personality and Social Psychology*, *52*, 861–870.

Glass, D.C. (1977). *Behavior patterns, stress, and coronary disease*. Hillsdale, NJ: Erlbaum Associates.

Goldstein, S., Gordon, J.R., & Marlatt, G.A. (1984, August). *Attributional processes and relapse following smoking cessation*. Paper presented at the 92nd Annual Convention of the American Psychological Association, Toronto, Canada.

Golin, S., Sweeney, P.D., & Schaeffer, D.E. (1981). The causality of causal attributions in depression: A cross-lagged panel correlational analysis. *Journal of Abnormal Psychology*, *90*, 14–22.

Gollwitzer, P.M., Earle, W.B., & Stephan, W.G. (1982). Affect as a determinant of egotism: Residual excitation and performance attributions. *Journal of Personality and Social Psychology*, *43*, 702–709.

Gottman, J.M. (1979). *Marital interaction*. New York: Academic Press.

Gould, R., & Sigall, H. (1977). The effects of empathy and outcome on attribution: An examination of the divergent perspective hypothesis. *Journal of Experimental Social Psychology*, *13*, 480–491.

Graham, S. (1984). Communicating sympathy and anger to black and white children: The cognitive (attributional) consequences of affective cues. *Journal of Personality and Social Psychology*, *47*, 40–54.

Graham, S., & Long, A. (1986). Race, class, and the attributional process. *Journal of Educational Psychology*, *78*, 4–13.

Graham, S., & Weiner, B. (1986). From an attributional theory of emotion to developmental psychology: A round-trip ticket? *Social Cognition*, *4*, 152–179.

Green, S.G., Lightfoot, M.A., Bandy, C., & Buchanan, D.R. (1985). A general model of the attribution process. *Basic and Applied Social Psychology*, *6*, 159–179.

Greenberg, J. (1980). Attentional focus and locus of performance causality as determinants of equity behavior. *Journal of Personality and Social Psychology*, *38*, 579–585.

Greenberg, J. (1983). *Difficult goal choice as a self-handicapping strategy*. Unpublished manuscript, Ohio State University, Columbus, Ohio.

Greenberg, J., Pyszczynski, T., & Solomon, S. (1982). The self-serving attributional bias: Beyond self-presentation. *Journal of Experimental Social Psychology*, *18*, 56–67.

Greene, D., & Lepper, M.R. (1974). Effects of extrinsic rewards on children's subsequent intrinsic interest. *Child Development*, *45*, 1141–1145.

Greenwald, A.G. (1980). The totalitarian ego: Fabrication and revision of personal history. *American Psychologist*, *35*, 603–618.

Grossarth-Maticek, R., Bastiaans, J., & Kanizer, D.T. (1985). Psychosocial factors as strong predictors of mortality from cancer, ischaemic heart disease and stroke: The Yugoslav prospective study. *Journal of Psychosomatic Research*, *29*, 167–176.

Guttentag, M., & Longfellow, C. (1978). Children's social attributions: Development and change. In C.B. Keasey (Ed.), *Nebraska symposium on motivation, 1977 (Vol. 25)* (pp. 305–342). Lincoln: University of Nebraska Press.

Hamilton, V.L. (1980). Intuitive psychologist or intuitive lawyer: Alternative models of the attribution process. *Journal of Personality and Social Psychology*, *39*, 767–772.

Hammen, C., & Cochran, S.D. (1981). Cognitive correlates of life stress and depression in college students. *Journal of Abnormal Psychology*, *90*, 23–27.

Hammen, C., & DeMayo, R. (1982). Cognitive correlates of teacher stress and depressive symptoms: Implications for attributional models of depression. *Journal of Abnormal Psychology*, *90*, 96–101.

Hansen, R.D. (1980). Commonsense attribution. *Journal of Personality and Social Psychology*, *39*, 996–1009.

Hansen, R.D. (1985). Cognitive economy and commonsense attribution processing. In J.H. Harvey & G. Weary (Eds.), *Attribution: Basic issues and applications* (pp. 65–86). Orlando, FL: Academic Press.

Hansen, R.D., & Donoghue, J.M. (1977). The power of consensus: Information derived from one's own and others' behavior. *Journal of Personality and Social Psychology*, *35*, 294–302.

Hansen, R.D., & Hall, C.A. (1985). Discounting and augmenting facilitative and inhibitory forces: The winner takes almost all. *Journal of Personality and Social Psychology*, *49*, 1482–1493.

Hansen, R.D., Hansen, C.H., & Crano, W.D. (in press). Sympathetic arousal, linguistic self-reference, and mere exposure: The consequences of directing attention to the self for the accessibility of self-states. *Journal of Experimental Social Psychology*.

Harackiewicz, J.M. Sansone, C., Blair, L.W., Epstein, J.A., & Manderlink, G. (1987). Attributional processes in behavior change and maintenance: Smoking cessation and continued abstinence. *Journal of Consulting and Clinical Psychology*, *55*, 372–378.

Harris, B. (1977). Developmental differences in the attribution of responsibility. *Developmental Psychology*, *13*, 257–265.

Harris, B. (1981). Developmental aspects of the attributional process. In J.H. Harvey & G. Weary, *Perspectives on attributional processes* (pp. 59–75). Dubuque, IA: Brown.

Harvey, J.H. (1989). People's naïve understandings of their close relationships: Attributional and personal construct perspectives. *International Journal of Personal Construct Psychology*, *2*, 37–49.

Harvey, J.H., Agostinelli, G., & Weber, A.L. (1989). Account-making and the formation of expectations about close relationships. *Review of Personality and Social Psychology*, *10*, 39–62.

Harvey, J.H., Arkin, R.M., Gleason, J.M., & Johnston, S. (1974). Effect of expected and observed outcome of an action on the differential causal attributions of actor and observer. *Journal of Personality*, *42*, 62–77.

Harvey, J.H., Bratt, A., & Lennox, R.D. (1987). The maturing interface of social–clinical–counseling psychology. *Journal of Social and Clinical Psychology*, *5*, 8–20.

Harvey, J.H., & Galvin, K.S. (1984). Clinical implications of attribution theory and research. *Clinical Psychology Review*, *4*, 15–33.

Harvey, J.H., Harris, B., & Barnes, R.D. (1975). Actor–observer differences in the perceptions of responsibility and freedom. *Journal of Personality and Social Psychology*, *32*, 22–28.

Harvey, J.H., Ickes, W., & Kidd, R.F. (Eds.). (1976). *New directions in attribution research (Vol. 1)*. Hillsdale, NJ: Erlbaum Associates.

Harvey, J.H., Town, J.P., & Yarkin, K.L. (1981). How fundamental is "the fundamental attribution error?" *Journal of Personality and Social Psychology*, *40*, 346–349.

Harvey, J.H., & Tucker, J.A. (1979). On problems with the cause–reason distinction in attribution theory. *Journal of Personality and Social Psychology*, *37*, 1441–1446.

Harvey, J.H., Turnquist, D.C., & Agostinelli, G. (1988). Identifying attributions in oral and written material. In C. Antaki (Eds.), *Analyzing lay explanation: A casebook of methods* (pp. 32–42). London: Sage.

Harvey, J.H., & Weary, G. (1981). *Perspectives on attributional processes*. Dubuque, IA: Brown.

Harvey, J.H., & Weary, G. (1984). Current issues in attribution theory and research. *Annual Review of Psychology*, *35*, 427–459.

Harvey, J.H., & Weary, G. (Eds.). (1985). *Attribution: Basic issues and applications*. Orlando, FL: Academic Press.

Harvey, J.H., Weber, A.L., Galvin, K.S., Huszti, H.C., & Garnick, N.N. (1986). Attribution and the termination of close relationships: A special focus on the account. In R. Gilmour & S. Duck (Eds.), *The emerging field of personal relationships* (pp. 189–201). Hillsdale, NJ: Erlbaum Associates.

Harvey, J.H., Wells, G.L., & Alvarez, M.D. (1978). Attribution in the context of conflict and separation in close relationships. In J.H. Harvey, W.J. Ickes, & R.F. Kidd (Eds.), *New directions in attribution research (Vol. 2)* (pp. 235–259). Hillsdale, NJ: Erlbaum Associates.

Harvey, J.H., Yarkin, K.L., Lightner, J.M., & Town, J.P. (1980). Unsolicited interpretation and recall of interpersonal events. *Journal of Personality and Social Psychology*, *38*, 551–568.

Hastie, R. (1981). Schematic principles in human memory. In E.T. Higgins, C.P. Herman, & M.P. Zanna (Eds.), *Social cognition: The Ontario symposium (Vol. 1)* (pp. 39–88). Hillsdale, NJ: Erlbaum Associates.

Hastie, R. (1983). Social inference. *Annual Review of Psychology*, *34*, 511–542.

Hastie, R. (1984). Causes and effects of causal attributions. *Journal of Personality and Social Psychology*, *46*, 44–56.

Hastie, R., & Kumar, P.A. (1979). Person memory: Personality traits as organizing principles in memory for behavior. *Journal of Personality and Social Psychology*, *37*, 25–38.

Hastie, R., & Park, B. (1986). The relationship between memory and judgment depends on whether the judgment task is memory-based or on-line. *Psychological Review*, *93*, 258–268.

Heerwagen, J.H., Beach, L.R., & Mitchell, T.R. (1985). Dealing with poor performance: Supervisor attributions and the cost of responding. *Journal of Applied Social Psychology*, *15*, 638–655.

Heider, F. (1944). Social perception and phenomenal causality. *Psychological Review*, *51*, 358–374.

Heider, F. (1958). *The psychology of interpersonal relations*. New York: John Wiley & Sons.

Heider, F. (1959). The function of the perceptual system. *Psychological Issues*, *1*, 35–52.

Hewstone, M. (Ed.). (1983). *Causal attribution: From cognitive processes to collective beliefs*. Oxford: Basil Blackwell.

Hewstone, M. (in press). *Causal attribution: From cognitive processes to collective beliefs*. Oxford: Basil Blackwell.

Hill, M.G., Weary, G., Hildebrand-Saints, L., & Elbin, S.D. (1985). Social comparison of causal understandings. In J.H. Harvey & G. Weary (Eds.), *Attribution: Basic issues and applications* (pp. 143–166). Orlando, FL: Academic Press.

Hill M.G., Weary, G., & Williams, J.P. (1986). Depression: A self-presentation formulation of depression. In R.F. Baumeister (Ed.), *Public self and private self* (pp. 213–240). New York: Springer-Verlag.

Hilton, D.J., & Slugoski, B.R. (1986). Knowledge-based causal attribution: The abnormal conditions focus model. *Journal of Personality and Social Psychology*, *93*, 75–88.

Himmelfarb, S., & Anderson, N.H. (1975). Integration-theory applied to opinion attribution. *Journal of Personality and Social Psychology*, *31*, 1064–1071.

Hiroto, D.S. (1974). Locus of control and learned helplessness. *Journal of Experimental Psychology*, *102*, 187–193.

Hiroto, D.S., & Seligman, M.E.P. (1975). Generality of learned helplessness in man. *Journal of Personality and Social Psychology*, *31*, 311–327.

Hoffman, M.L. (1970). Moral development. In P.H. Mussen (Ed.), *Carmichael's manual of child psychology (3rd ed., Vol. 2)* (pp. 261–359). New York: Wiley.

Holtzworth-Munroe, A., & Jacobson, N.J. (1985). Causal attributions of married couples. *Journal of Personality and Social Psychology*, *48*, 1398–1412.

Ickes, W. (in press). Using the dyadic interaction paradigm. *Review of Personality and Social Psychology*.

Ickes, W.J., & Kidd, R.F. (1976). Attributional analysis of helping behavior. In J.H. Harvey, W.J. Ickes, & R.F. Kidd (Eds.), *New directions in attribution research (Vol. 1)* (pp. 311–334). Hillsdale, NJ: Erlbaum Associates.

Imamoglu, E.O. (1976). Children's awareness and usage of intention cues. *Child Development*, *46*, 39–45.

Ingram, R.E., Kendall, P.C., Smith, T.W., Donnell, C., & Ronan, K. (1987). Cognitive specificity in emotional distress. *Journal of Personality and Social Psychology*, *53*, 734–742.

Ittelson, W.H., Proshansky, H.M., Rivlin, L.G., & Winkel, G.H. (1974). *Introduction to environmental psychology*. New York: Holt, Rinehart, & Winston.

Jacobson, N.S., Follette, W.C., & McDonald, D.W. (1982). Reactivity to positive and negative behavior in distressed and nondistressed married couples. *Journal of Consulting and Clinical Psychology*, 706–714.

Jacobson, N.S., McDonald, D.E., Follette, W.C., & Berley, R.A. (1985). Attributional processes in distressed and nondistressed married couples. *Cognitive Therapy and Research, 9*, 35–50.

Janoff-Bulman, R. (1978, August). *Self-blame in rape victims: Control-maintenance strategy.* Paper presented at the American Psychological Association meeting, Toronto, Canada.

Janoff-Bulman, R. (1979). Characterological versus behavioral self-blame: Inquiries into depression and rape. *Journal of Personality and Social Psychology, 37*, 1798–1809.

Janoff-Bulman, R. (1982). Esteem and control bases of blame: "Adaptive" strategies for victims versus observers. *Journal of Personality, 50*, 180–192.

Janoff-Bulman, R., & Frieze, I.H. (1983). A theoretical perspective for understanding reactions to victimization. *Journal of Social Issues, 39*, 1–17.

Janoff-Bulman, R., & Wortman, C.B. (1977). Attributions of blame and coping in the "real world": Severe accident victims react to their lot. *Journal of Personality and Social Psychology, 35*, 351–363.

Jaspars, J., Fincham, F., & Hewstone, M. (Eds.). (1983). *Attribution theory and research: Conceptual, developmental, and social dimensions.* London: Academic Press.

Jeffrey, D.B. (1974). A comparison of the effects of external control and self-control on the modification and maintenance of weight. *Journal of Abnormal Psychology, 83*, 404–410.

Johnson, W.G., Ross, J.M., & Mastria, M.A. (1977). Delusional behavior: An attributional analysis of development and modification. *Journal of Abnormal Psychology, 86*, 421–426.

Jones, E.E. (1979). The rocky road from acts to dispositions. *American Psychologist, 34*, 107–117.

Jones, E.E. (1987). Retrospective review of F. Heider's *The Psychology of Interpersonal Relations:* The seer who found attributional wisdom in naivety. *Contemporary Psychology, 32*, 213–216.

Jones, E.E., & Berglas, S. (1978). Control of attributions about the self through self-handicapping strategies: The appeal of alcohol and the role of underachievement. *Personality and Social Psychology Bulletin, 4*, 200–206.

Jones, E.E., & Davis, K.E. (1965). From acts to dispositions: The attribution process in person perception. In L. Berkowitz (Ed.), *Advances in experimental social psychology (Vol. 2)* (pp. 219–266). New York: Academic Press.

Jones, E.E., Davis, K.E., & Gergen, K.J. (1961). Role playing variations and their informational value for person perception. *Journal of Abnormal and Social Psychology, 63*, 302–310.

Jones, E.E., Farina, A., Hastorf, A., Markus, H., Miller, D., & Scott, R.A. (1984). *Social stigma: The psychology of marked relationships.* San Francisco: W.H. Freeman.

Jones, E.E., & Harris, V.A. (1967). The attribution of attitudes. *Journal of Experimental Social Psychology, 3*, 1–24.

Jones, E.E., Kanouse, D.E., Kelley, H.H., Nisbett, R.E., Valins, S., & Weiner,

B. (Eds.). (1972). *Attribution: Perceiving the causes of behavior.* Morristown, NJ: General Learning Press.

Jones. E.E., & Kelley, H.H. (1978). A conversation with Edward Jones and Harold H. Kelley. In J.H. Harvey, W.J., Ickes, & R.F. Kidd (Eds.), *New directions in attribution research (Vol. 2)* (pp. 371–388). Hillsdale, NJ: Erlbaum Associates.

Jones, E.E., & McGillis, D. (1976). Correspondent inferences and the attribution cube: A comparative reappraisal. In J.H. Harvey, W.J. Ickes, R.F. Kidd (Eds.), *New directions in attribution research (Vol. 1)* (pp. 389–420). Hillsdale, NJ: Erlbaum Associates.

Jones, E.E., & Nisbett, R.E. (1972). The actor and the observer: Divergent perceptions of the causes of behavior. In E.E. Jones, D.E. Kanouse, H.H. Kelley, R.E. Nisbett, S. Valins, & B. Weiner (Eds.), *Attribution: Perceiving the causes of behavior* (pp. 79–94). Morristown, NJ: General Learning Press.

Jones, E.E., & Sigall, H. (1971). The bogus pipeline: A new paradigm for measuring affect and attitude. *Psychological Bulletin*, 76, 349–364.

Jones, E.E., Worchel, S., Goethals, G.R., & Grumet, J.F. (1971). Prior expectancy and behavioral extremity as determinants of attitude attribution. *Journal of Experimental Social Psychology*, 7, 59–80.

Jones, R.A., Linder. D.E., Kiesler, C.A., Zanna, M., & Brehm, J. (1968). Internal states or external stimuli: Observers' attitude judgments and the dissonance theory–self-persuasion controversy. *Journal of Experimental Social Psychology*, 4, 247–269.

Karniol, R. (1978). Children's use of intention cues in evaluating behavior. *Psychological Bulletin*, 85, 76–85.

Karniol, R., & Ross, M. (1976). The development of causal attributions in social perception. *Journal of Personality and Social Psychology*, 34, 455–464.

Kassin, S.M. (1979). Consensus information, prediction, and causal attribution: A review of the literature and issues. *Journal of Personality and Social Psychology*, 37, 1966–1981.

Kassin, S.M., & Baron, R.M. (1985). Basic determinants of attribution and social perception. In J.H. Harvey & G. Weary (Eds.), *Attribution: Basic issues and applications* (pp. 37–64). Orlando, FL: Academic Press.

Kassin, S., & Lepper, M.R. (1984). Oversufficient and insufficient justification effects: Cognitive and behavioral development. In J. Nicholls (Ed.), *Advances in Motivation and Achievement (Vol. 3)* (pp. 73–106). Greenwich, CT: JAI Press.

Keasey, C.B. (1978). Children's developing awareness and usage of intentionality and motives. In C.B. Keasey (Ed.), *Nebraska symposium on motivation, 1977 (Vol. 25)* (pp. 219–260). Lincoln: University of Nebraska Press.

Kelley, H.H. (1967). Attribution theory in social psychology. In D. Levine (Ed.), *Nebraska symposium on motivation (Vol. 15)* (pp. 192–240). Lincoln: University of Nebraska Press.

Kelley, H.H. (1971). *Attribution in social interaction.* Morristown, NJ: General Learning Corporation.

Kelley, H.H. (1972a). Causal schemata and the attribution process. In E.E. Jones, D.E. Kanouse, H.H. Kelley, R.E. Nisbett, S. Valins, & B. Weiner (Eds.), *Attribution: Perceiving the causes of behavior* (pp. 151–174). Morristown, NJ: General Learning Press.

Kelley, H.H. (1972b). Attribution in social interaction. In E.E. Jones, D.E. Kanouse, H.H. Kelley, R.E. Nisbett, S. Valins, & B. Weiner (Eds.), *Attribution: Perceiving the causes of behavior* (pp. 1–26). Morristown, NJ: General Learning Press.

Kelley, H.H. (1973). The process of causal attribution. *American Psychologist, 28*, 107–128.

Kelley, H.H. (1978). A conversation with Edward E. Jones and Harold H. Kelley. In J.H. Harvey W.J. Ickes, R.F. Kidd (Eds.), *New directions in attribution research (Vol. 2)* (pp. 371–388). Hillsdale, NJ: Erlbaum Associates.

Kelley, H.H. (1979). *Personal relationships: Their structures and processes.* Hillsdale, NJ: Erlbaum Associates.

Kelley, H.H. (1983). Epilogue: Perceived causal structures. In J. Jaspars, F. Fincham, & M. Hewstone (Eds.), *Attribution theory: Essays and experiments* (pp. 320–335). London: Academic Press.

Kelley, H.H., Berscheid, E., Christensen, A., Harvey, J.H., Huston, T., Levinger, G., McClintock, E., Peplau, A., & Peterson, D. (1983). *Close relationships.* San Francisco: Freeman.

Kelley, H.H., & Michela, J.L. (1980). Attribution theory and research. *Annual of Review of Psychology, 31*, 457–501.

Kelley, K., & Forsyth, D.R. (1984, April). *Attribution–affect linkages after success and failure.* Paper presented at the annual meeting of the Eastern Psychological Association, Baltimore, MD.

Kellogg, R., & Baron, R.S. (1975). Attribution theory, insomnia, and the reverse placebo effect: A reversal of Storms and Nisbett's findings. *Journal of Personality and Social Psychology, 32*, 231–236.

Kelly, G.A. (1955). *The psychology of personal constructs.* New York: Norton.

Kent, R.N., Wilson, G.T., & Nelson, R. (1972). Effects of false heart-rate feedback on avoidance behavior: An investigation of "cognitive desensitization." *Behavior Therapy, 3*, 1–6.

Kiecolt-Glaser, J.K., Garner, W., Speicher, C.E., Penn, G.M., Holliday, J.E., & Glaser, R. (1984). Psychosocial modifiers of immunocompetence in medical students. *Psychosomatic Medicine, 46*, 7–14.

Kiecolt-Glaser, J.K., Glaser, R., Williger, D., Stout, J., Messick, G., Sheppard, J., Ricker, D., Romisher, S.C., Brener, W., Bonnell, G., & Donnerberg, R. (1985). Psychosocial enhancement of immunocompetence in a geriatric population. *Health Psychology, 4*, 25–41.

Kiecolt-Glaser, J.K., & Williams, D.A. (1987). Self-blame, compliance, and distress among burn patients. *Journal of Personality and Social Psychology, 53*, 187–193.

King, M. (1971). The development of some intention concepts in young children. *Child Development, 42*, 1145–1152.

Klein, D.C., Fencil-Morse, E., & Seligman, M.E.P. (1976). Learned helplessness, depression, and the attribution of failure. *Journal of Personality and Social Psychology, 33*, 508–516.

Kinger, E. (1977). *Meaning and void.* Minneapolis: University of Minnesota Press.

Kolditz, T.A., & Arkin, R.M. (1982). An impression management interpretation of the self-handicapping strategy. *Journal of Personality and Social Psychology, 43*, 492–502.

Kopel, S., & Arkowitz, H. (1975). The role of attribution and self-perception in behavior change: Implications for behavior therapy. *Genetic Psychology Monographs*, *92*, 175–212.

Kovenglioglu, G., & Greenhaus, J.H. (1978). Causal attributions, expectations, and task performance. *Journal of Applied Psychology*, *63*, 698–705.

Kruglanski, A.W. (1975). The endogenous–exogenous partition in attribution theory. *Psychological Review*, *82*, 387–406.

Kruglanski, A.W. (1979). Causal explanation, teleological explanation: On radical particularism in attribution theory. *Journal of Personality and Social Psychology*, *37*, 1447–1457.

Kruglanski, A.W., Hamel, I.Z., Maides, S.A., & Schwartz, J.M. (1978). Attribution theory as a special case of lay epistemology. In J.H. Harvey, W.J. Ickes, & R.F. Kidd (Eds.), *New directions in attribution research (Vol. 2)* (pp. 299–333). Hillsdale, NJ: Erlbaum Associates.

Kuiper, N.A. (1978). Depression and causal attributions for success and failure. *Journal of Personality and Social Psychology*, *36*, 236–246.

Kulik, J.A., & Taylor, S.E. (1980). Effects of sample-based versus self-based consensus information. *Journal of Personality and Social Psychology*, *38*, 871–878.

Kyle, S.O., & Falbo, T. (1985). Relationships between marital stress and attributional preferences for own and spouse behavior. *Journal of Social and Clinical Psychology*, *3*, 339–351.

Laing, R.D. (1961). *Self and others*. New York: Penguin Books.

Laing, R.D., Phillipson, H., & Lee, A.R. (1966). *International perception*. New York: Springer.

Lassiter, D., Stone, J.I., & Rogers, S.L. (1988). Memorial consequences of variation in behavior perception. *Journal of Experimental Social Psychology*, *24*, 222–239.

Lau, R.R., & Russell, S. (1980). Attributions in the sports pages. *Journal of Personality and Social Psychology*, *39*, 29–38.

Lazarus, R.S. (1966). *Psychological stress and the coping process*. New York: McGraw-Hill.

Leary, M.R., & Miller, R.S. (1986). *Social psychology and dysfunctional behavior: Origins, diagnosis, and treatment*. New York: Springer-Verlåg.

Leggett, E.L., & Dweck, C.S. (1986). *Goals and inference rules: Sources of causal judgments*. Manuscript submitted for publication.

Lepper, M.R. (1983a). Social-control processes and the internalization of social values: An attributional perspective. In E.T. Higgins, D.N. Ruble, & W.W. Hartup (Eds.), *Social cognition and social development* (pp. 294–330). New York: Cambridge.

Lepper, M.R. (1983b). Extrinsic reward and intrinsic motivation: Implications for the classroom. In S.M. Levine & M.C. Wang (Eds.), *Teacher and student perceptions: Implications for learning* (pp. 281–317). Hillsdale, NJ: Erlbaum Associates.

Lepper, M.R., Greene, D., & Nisbett, R.E. (1973). Undermining children's intrinsic interest with extrinsic rewards: A test of the "overjustification" hypothesis. *Journal of Personality and Social Psychology*, *28*, 129–137.

Lepper, M.R., Sagotsky, G., Dafoe, J.L., & Greene, D. (1982). Consequences of superfluous social constraints: Effects on young children's social inferences and subsequent intrinsic interest. *Journal of Personality and Social Psychology*, *42*, 57–65.

Lerner, M.J. (1965). Evaluation of performance as a function of performer's reward and attractiveness. *Journal of Personality and Social Psychology*, *1*, 355–360.

Lerner, M.J., & Miller, D.T. (1978). Just world research and the attribution process: Looking back and ahead. *Psychological Bulletin*, *85*, 1030–1051.

Leslie, A.M. (1982). The perception of causality in infants. *Perception*, *11*, 173–186.

Leventhal, H., Brown D., Shacham, S., & Engquist, G. (1979). Effects of preparatory information about sensations: Threat of pain, and attention on cold pressor distress. *Journal of Personality and Social Psychology*, *37*, 688–714.

Livesley, W.J., & Bromley, D.B. (1973). *Person perception in childhood and adolescence*. London: Wiley.

Lloyd, S.A., & Cate, R. (1985). Attributions associated with significant turning points in premarital relationship development and dissolution. *Journal of Social and Personal Relationships*, *2*, 419–436.

Locke, D., & Pennington, D. (1982). Reasons and other causes: Their role in the attribution process. *Journal of Personality and Social Psychology*, *42*, 212–223.

London, H., & Nisbett, R.E. (Eds.). (1974). *Cognitive alterations of feeling states*. Chicago: Aldine.

Lowery, B.J., Jacobson, B.S., & Murphy, B.B. (1983). An exploratory investigation of causal thinking of arthritics. *Nursing Research*, *32*, 157–162.

Lowery, C.R., Denney, D.R., & Storms, M.D. (1979). Insomnia: A comparison of the effects of pill attributions and nonpejorative self-attributions. *Cognitive Therapy and Research*, *3*, 161–164.

Madden, M.E., & Janoff-Bulman, R. (1983). Blame, control, and marital satisfaction: Wives' attributions for conflict in marriage. *Journal of Marriage and the Family*, *44*, 663–674.

Maier, S.F., & Seligman, M.E.P. (1976). Learned helplessness: Theory and evidence. *Journal of Experimental Psychology*, *105*, 3–46.

Major, B. (1980). Information acquisition and attribution processes. *Journal of Personality and Social Psychology*, *39*, 1010–1023.

Marshall, G.D., & Zimbardo, P.G. (1979). Affective consequences of inadequately explained physiological arousal. *Journal of Personality and Social Psychology*, *37*, 970–988.

Maslach, C. (1979). Negative emotional biasing of unexplained arousal. *Journal of Personality and Social Psychology*, *37*, 953–969.

Matthews, K.A., & Haynes, S.G. (1986). Type A behavior pattern and coronary disease risk: Update and critical evaluation. *American Journal of Epidemiology*, *123*, 923–960.

Matthews, S.H. (1986). *Friendship through the life course: Oral biographies in old age*. Beverly Hills, CA: Sage.

McArthur, L.Z. (1972). The how and what of why: Some determinants and consequences of causal attribution. *Journal of Personality and Social Psychology*, *22*, 171–193.

McArthur, L.Z. (1980). Illusory causation and illusory correlation: Two epistemological accounts. *Personality and Social Psychology Bulletin*, *6*, 507–519.

McArthur, L.Z. (1981). What grabs you? The role of attention in impression formation and causal attribution. In E.T. Higgins, C.P. Herman, & M.P. Zanna (Eds.), *Social cognition: The Ontario symposium (Vol. 1)* (pp. 201–246). Hillsdale, NJ: Erlbaum Associates.

McArthur, L.Z., & Baron, R.M. (1983). Toward an ecological theory of social perception. *Psychological Review*, *90*, 215–238.

McFarland, C., & Ross, M. (1982). Impact of causal attributions on affective reactions to success and failure. *Journal of Personality and Social Psychology*, *43*, 937–946.

McFarland, C., & Ross, M. (1987). The relation between current impressions and memories of self and dating partners. *Journal of Personality and Social Psychology*, *13*, 228–238.

McMillan, J.H., & Forsyth, D.R. (1983). Attribution–affect relationships following classroom performance. *Contemporary Educational Psychology*, *8*, 109–118.

Mead, G.H. (1934). *Mind, self, and society*. Chicago: University of Chicago Press.

Meichenbaum, D. (1977). *Cognitive–behavior modification: An integrative approach*. New York: Plenum.

Mendelson, R., & Schultz, T.R. (1976). Covariation and temporal contiguity as principles of causal inference in young children. *Journal of Experimental Child Psychology*, *33*, 408–412.

Meyer, C.B., & Taylor, S.E. (1986). Adjustment to rape. *Journal of Personality and Social Psychology*, *50*, 1226–1234.

Meyer, J.P., & Mulherin, A. (1980). From attribution to helping: An analysis of the mediating effects of affect and expectancy. *Journal of Personality and Social Psychology*, *39*, 201–210.

Meyer, W.U. (1970). *Selbstverantworklichkeit und Leistungsmotivation*. Unpublished doctoral dissertation, Ruhr-Universität, Bochum, Germany. [In B. Weiner (1986), *An attributional theory of motivation and emotion*. New York: Springer-Verlag.]

Meyerowitz, B.E. (1980). Psychosocial correlates of breast cancer and its treatments. *Psychological Bulletin*, *87*, 108–131.

Michela, & Wood, J.V. (1986). Causal attributions in health and illness. In P.H. Kendall (Ed.), *Advances in cognitive–behavioral research and therapy (Vol. 5)* (pp. 179–235). New York: Academic Press.

Michotte, A. (1963). *The perception of causality*. London: Methuen.

Miller, D.T., & Norman, A. (1975). Actor–observer differences in perceptions of effective control. *Journal of Personality and Social Psychology*, *31*, 502–515.

Miller, D.T., & Porter, C.A. (1983). Self-blame in victims of violence. *Journal of Social Issues*, *39*, 139–152.

Miller, D.T., & Ross, M. (1975). Self-serving biases in the attribution of causality: Fact or fiction? *Psychological Bulletin*, *82*, 213–225.

Miller, J.G. (1984). Culture and the development of everyday social explanation. *Journal of Personality and Social Psychology*, *46*, 961–978.

Miller, I., Klee, S., & Norman, W. (1982). Depressed and nondepressed inpatients' cognitions of hypothetical events, experimental tasks, and stressful life events. *Journal of Abnormal Psychology*, *91*, 78–81.

Miller, I.W., & Norman, W.H. (1979). Learned helplessness in humans: A review and attribution-theory model. *Psychological Bulletin*, *86*, 93–118.

Miller, R.L., Brickman, P., & Bolen, D. (1975). Attribution versus persuasion as a means for modifying behavior. *Journal of Personality and Social Psychology*, *31*, 430–441.

Mills, J. (1967). Comment on Bem's "Self-perception: An alternative interpretation of cognitive dissonance phenomena." *Psychological Review*, *74*, 535.

Mirels, H.L. (1980). The avowal of responsibility for good and bad outcomes: The effects of generalized self-serving biases. *Personality and Social Psychology Bulletin, 6*, 299–306.

Monson, T.C., & Snyder, M. (1977). Actors, observers, and the attribution process: Toward a reconceptualization. *Journal of Experimental Social Psychology, 13*, 89–111.

Montgomery, R.L., & Haemmerlie, F.M. (1986). Self-perception theory and the reduction of heterosocial anxiety. *Journal of Social and Clinical Psychology, 4*, 503–512.

Murstein, B.I., & Beck, G.D. (1972). Person perception, marriage adjustment and social desirability. *Journal of Consulting and Clinical Psycology, 39*, 396–403.

Newman, H. (1981). Communication within ongoing intimate relationships: An attribution perspective. *Personality and Social Psychology Bulletin, 7*, 59–70.

Newtson, D. (1973). Attribution and the unit of perception of ongoing behavior. *Journal of Personality and Social Psychology, 10*, 28–38.

Newtson, D. (1974). Dispositional inference from effects of actions: Effects chosen and effects foregone. *Journal of Experimental Social Psychology, 10*, 489–496.

Newtson, D. (1976). Foundations of attribution: The perception of ongoing behavior. In J.H. Harvey, W.J. Ickes, & R.F. Kidd (Eds.), *New directions in attribution research (Vol. 1)* (pp. 223–248). Hillsdale, NJ: Elrbaum Associates.

Newtson, D.L., Engquist, G., & Bois, J. (1977). The objective basis of behavior units. *Journal of Personality and Social Psychology, 35*, 847–862.

Nicholls, J.G. (1975). Causal attributions and other achievement-related cognitions: Effects of task outcome, attainment value, and sex. *Journal of Personality and Social Psychology, 31*, 379–387.

Nicholls, J.G. (1976). Effort is virtuous, but it's better to have ability: Evaluative responses to perceptions of effort and ability. *Journal of Research in Personality, 10*, 306–315.

Nisbett, R.E., & Borgida, E. (1975). Attribution and the psychology of prediction. *Journal of Personality and Social Psychology, 32*, 932–943.

Nisbett, R.E., Caputo, C., Legant, P., & Marecek, J. (1973). Behavior as seen by the actor and as seen by the observer. *Journal of Personality and Social psychology, 27*, 154–164.

Nisbett, R.E., & Ross, L. (1980). *Human inference: Strategies and shortcomings of social judgment.* Englewood Cliffs, NJ: Prentice-Hall.

Nisbett, R.E., & Schachter, S. (1966). Cognitive manipulation of pain. *Journal of Experimental Social Psychology, 2*, 227–236.

Nisbett, R.E., & Wilson, T.D. (1977). Telling more than we can know: Verbal reports on mental processes. *Psychological Review, 84*, 231–259.

Noel, J.G., Forsyth, D.R., & Kelley, K.N. (1987). Improving the performance of failing students by overcoming their self-serving attributional biases. *Basic and Applied Social Psychology, 8*, 151–162.

Nolen-Hoeksema, S., Girgus, J.S., & Seligman, M.E.P. (1986). Learned helplessness in children: A longitudinal study of depression, achievement, and explanatory style. *Journal of Personality and Social Psychology, 51*, 435–442.

Nummedal, S.G., & Bass, S.C. (1976). Effects of the salience of intention and consequence on children's moral judgments. *Developmental Psychology, 12*, 475–476.

Olson, J.M. (1988). Misattribution, preparatory information, and speech anxiety. *Journal of Personality and Social Psychology, 54*, 758–767.

Olson, J.M., & Ross, M. (1985). Attribution research: Past contributions, current trends, and future prospects. In J.H. Harvey & G. Weary (Eds.), *Attribution: Basic issues and applications* (pp. 283–312). Orlando, FL: Academic Press.

Olson, J.M., & Ross, M. (in press). False feedback about placebo effectiveness: Consequences for the misattribution of speech anxiety. *Journal of Experimental Social Psychology*.

Orvis, B.R., Cunningham, J.D., & Kelley, H.H. (1975). A closer examination of causal inference: The roles of consensus, distinctiveness, and consistency information. *Journal of Personality and Social Psychology*, *32*, 605–616.

Orvis, B.R., Kelley, H.H., & Butler, D. (1976). Attributional conflict in young couples. In J.H. Harvey, W.J. Ickes, & R.F. Kidd (Eds.), *New directions in attribution research (Vol. 1)* (pp. 353–386). Hillsdale, NJ: Erlbaum Associates.

Overmier, J.B., & Seligman, M.E.P. (1967). Effects of inescapable shock upon subsequent escape and avoidance learning. *Journal of Comparative and Physiological Psychology*, *63*, 23–33.

Passer, M.W., Kelley, H.H., & Michela, J.L. (1978). Multidimensional scaling of the causes for negative interpersonal behavior. *Journal of Personality and Social Psychology*, *36*, 951–962.

Peterson, C. (1980). Attribution in the sports pages: An archival investigation of the covariation hypothesis. *Social Psychology Quarterly*, *43*, 136–141.

Peterson, C., Luborsky, L. & Seligman, M.E.P. (1983). Attributions and depressive mood shifts: A case study using the symptom–context method. *Journal of Abnormal Psychology*, *92*, 96–103.

Peterson, C., & Seligman, M.E.P. (1981). Helplessness and attributional style in depression. *Tiddsskrift for Norsk Psykologforening*, *18*, 3–18, 53–59.

Peterson, C., & Seligman, M.E.P. (1983). Learned helplessness and victimization. *Journal of Social Issues*, *2*, 103–116.

Peterson, C., & Seligman, M.E.P. (1984). Causal explanations as a risk factor for depression: Theory and evidence. *Psychological Review*, *91*, 347–374.

Peterson, C., Semmel, S., von Baeyer, C., Abramson, L.Y., Metalsky, G.I., & Seligman, M.E.P. (1982). The attribution style questionnaire. *Cognitive Therapy and Research*, *6*, 287–299

Peterson, C., & Villanova, P. (1988). An expanded attributional style questionnaire. *Journal of Abnormal Psychology*, *97*, 87–89

Piaget, J. (1932). *The moral judgment of the child.* New York: Harcourt, Brace.

Pittman, T.S., & D'Agostino, P.R. (1985). Motivation and attribution: The effects of control deprivation on subsequent information processing. In J.H. Harvey & G. Weary (Eds.), *Attribution: Basic issues and applications* (pp. 000–000). New York: Academic Press.

Pittman, T.S., & Pittman, N.L. (1980). Deprivation of control and the attribution process. *Journal of Personality and Social Psychology*, *39*, 377–389

Powers, S., Douglas, P., Cool, B.A., & Gose, K.F. (1985). Achievement motivation and attributions for success and failure. *Psychological Reports*, *57*, 751–754.

Powers, S., & Wagner, M.J. (1983). Attributions for success and failure of Hispanic and Anglo high school students. *Journal of Instructional Psychology*, *19*, 171–176.

Powers, S., & Wagner, M.J. (1984). Attributions for school achievement of middle school students. *Journal of Early Adolescence*, *4*, 215–222.

Pryor, J.P., Rholes, W.S., Ruble, D.N., & Kriss, M. (1984). Developmental analysis of salience and discounting in social attribution. *Representative Research in Social Psychology*, *14*, 30–40.

Pyszczynski, T.A., & Greenberg, J. (1981). Role of disconfirmed expectancies in the instigation of attributional processing. *Journal of Personality and Social Psychology*, *40*, 31–38.

Quattrone, G.A. (1982). Overattribution and unit formation: When behavior engulfs the person. *Journal of Personality and Social Psychology*, *42*, 593–607.

Rapps, C.S., Peterson, C., Reinhard, K.E., Abramson, L.Y., & Seligman, M.E.P. (1982). Attributional style among depressed patients. *Journal of Abnormal Psychology*, *91*, 102–108.

Raush, H.J., Barry, W.A., Hertel, R.K., & Swain, M.A. (1974). *Communication, conflict, and marriage*. San Francisco: Jossey-Bass.

Read, S.J. (1984). Analogical reasoning in social judgment: The importance of causal theories. *Journal of Personality and Social Psychology*, *46*, 14–25.

Read, S.J. (1987). Constructing causal scenarios: A knowledge structure approach to causal reasoning. *Journal of Personality and Social Psychology*, *52*, 288–302.

Reeder, G.D. (1985). Implicit relations between dispositions and behavior: Effects on dispositional attribution. In J.H. Harvey & G. Weary (Eds.), *Attribution: Basic issues and applications* (pp. 87–116). Orlando, FL: Academic Press.

Reeder, G.D., & Brewer, M.B. (1979). A schematic model of dispositional attribution in interpersonal perception. *Psychological Review*, *86*, 61–79.

Reeder, G.D., & Fulks, J.L. (1980). When actions speak louder than words: Implicational schemata and the attribution of ability. *Journal of Experimental Social Psychology*, *16*, 33–46.

Reeder, G.D., Henderson, D.J., & Sullivan, J.J. (1982). From dispositions to behaviors: The flip side of attribution. *Journal of Research in Personality*, *16*, 355–375.

Reeder, G.D., Messick, D.M., & Van Avermaet, E. (1977). Dimensional asymmetry in attributional inference. *Journal of Experimental Social Psychology*, *13*, 46–57.

Reeder, G.D., & Spores, J.M. (1983, May). *Individual differences in the attitude attribution paradigm*. Paper presented at the meeting of the Midwestern Psychological Association, Chicago, IL.

Regan, D.T. (1978). Attributional aspects of interpersonal attraction. In J.H. Harvey, W.J. Ickes, & R.F. Kidd (Eds.), *New directions in attribution research (Vol. 2)* (pp. 212–235). Hillsdale, NJ: Erlbaum Associates.

Regan, D.T., & Totten, J. (1975). Empathy and attribution: Turning observes into actors. *Journal of Personality and Social Psychology*, *32*, 850–856.

Rehm, L.P. (1981). A self-control therapy program for treatment of depression. In J.F. Clarkin & H.I. Glazer (Eds.), *Depression: Behavioral and directive intervention strategies* (pp. 68–111). New York: Garland Press.

Reisenzein, R. (1983). The Schachter theory of emotion: Two decades later. Psychological Bulletin, *94*, 239–264.

Reisenzein, R., & Gattinger, E. (1982). Salience of arousal as a mediator of misattribution of transferred excitation. *Motivation and Emotion*, *6*, 315–328.

Review Panel on Coronary-Prone Behavior and Coronary Heart Disease. (1981). Coronary-prone behavior and coronary heart disease: A critical review. *Circulation*, *63*, 1199–1215.

Rhodewalt, F. (1984). Self-improvement, self-attribution, and the Type A coronary-prone behavior pattern. *Journal of Personality and Social Psychology*, *47*, 662–670.

Rhodewalt, F., & Davision, J. (1984). *Self-handicapping and subsequent performance: The role of outcome valence and attributional certainty.* Unpublished manuscript, University of Utah, Salt Lake City.

Rhodewalt, F., & Marcroft, M. (1988). Type A behavior and diabetic control: Implications of psychological reactance for health outcomes. *Journal of Applied Social Psychology 18*, 139–159.

Rhodewalt, F., & Strube, M.J. (1985). A self-attribution–reactance model of recovery from injury in Type A individuals. *Journal of Applied Social Psychology*, *15*, 300–344.

Rholes, W.S., & Walters, J. (1982). Schematic patterns of causal evidence. *Child Development*, *53*, 1046–1057.

Rich, M.C. (1979). Verbal reports on mental processes: Issues of accuracy and awareness. *Journal for the Theory of Social Behavior*, *9*, 29–37.

Riess, M., Rosenfeld, R., Melburg, V., & Tedeschi, J.T. (1981). Self-serving attributions: Biased private perceptions and distorted public descriptions. *Journal of Personality and Social Psychology*, *41*, 224–231.

Rosenbaum, R.M. (1972). *A dimensional analysis of the perceived causes of success and failure.* Unpublished doctoral dissertation, University of California, Los Angeles. [Cited in B. Weiner (1979), A theory of motivation for some classroom experiences. *Journal of Educational Psychology*, *71*, 3–25.]

Rosenblatt, P.C. (1983). *Bitter, biter tears.* Minneapolis: Univesity of Minnesota Press.

Rosenfield, D., & Stephan, W.G. (1978). Sex differences in attributions for sex-typed tasks. *Journal of Personality*, *46*, 244–259.

Ross, L. (1977). The intuitive psychologist and his shortcomings: Distortions in the attribution process. In L. Berkowitz (Ed.), *Advances in experimental social psychology (Vol, 10)* (pp. 173–220). New York: Academic Press.

Ross, L., Rodin, J., & Zimbardo, P.G. (1969). Toward an attribution therapy: The reduction of fear through induced cognitive–emotional misattribution. *Journal of Personality and Social Psychology*, *12*, 279–288.

Ross, M. (1975). Salience of reward and intrinsic motivation. *Journal of Personality and Social Psychology*, *32*, 245–254.

Ross, M., & Fletcher, G.J.O. (1985). Attribution and social perception. In G. Lindzey & E. Aronson (Eds.), *The handbook of social psychology* (pp. 73–122). New York: Random House.

Ross, M., & Olson, J.M. (1981). An expectancy–attribution model of the effects of placebos. *Psychological Review*, *88*, 408–437.

Ross, M., & Sicoly, F. (1979). Egocentric biases in availability and attribution. *Journal of Personality and Social Psychology*, *37*, 322–336.

Roth, S., & Bootzin, R.R. (1974). Effects of experimentally induced expectancies of external control: An investigation of learned helplessness. *Journal of Personality and Social Psychology*, *29*, 253–264.

Roth, S., & Kubal, L. (1975). Effects of non-contingent reinforcement on tasks of differing importance: Facilitation and learned helplessness. *Journal of Personality and Social Psychology*, *32*, 680–691.

Rothbaum, F., Weisz, J.R., & Snyder, S.S. (1982). Changing the world and changing the self: A two-process model of perceived control. *Journal of Personality and Social Psychology*, *42*, 5–37.

Rotter, J.B. (1966). Generalized expectancies for internal versus external control of reinforcement. *Psychological Monographs*, *80*, (1, Whole No. 609).

Ruble, D.N., & Feldman, N.S. (1976). Order of consensus, distinctiveness, and consistency information and causal attributions. *Journal of Personality and Social Psychology*, *34*, 930–937.

Ruble, D.N., Feldman, N.S., Higgins, E.T., & Karlovac, M. (1979). Focus of causality and the use of information in the development of causal attributions. *Journal of Personality*, *49*, 595–614.

Russell, D. (1982). The causal dimension scale: A measure of how individuals perceive causes. *Journal of Personality and Social Psychology*, *42*, 1137–1145.

Russell, D., Lenel, J., Spicer, C., Miller, J., Albrecht, J., & Rose, J. (1985). Evaluating the handicapped: An attributional analysis. *Personality and Social Psychology Bulletin*, *11*, 23–31.

Russell, D., McAuley, E., & Tarico, V. (1987). Measuring causal attributions for success and failure: A comparison of methodologies for assessing causal dimensions. *Personality and Social Psychology*, *53*, 1248–1257.

Schachter, S. (1964). The interaction of cognitive and physiological determinants of emotional state. In L. Berkowitz (Ed.), *Advances in experimental social psychology* (pp. 49–80). New York: Academic Press.

Schachter, S., & Singer, J.E. (1962). Cognitive, social, and physiological determinants of emotional state. *Psychological Review*, *69*, 379–399.

Schachter, S., & Singer, J.E. (1979). Comments on the Maslach and Marshall–Zimbardo experiments. *Journal of Personality and Social Psychology*, *37*, 989–995.

Schank, R., & Abelson, R. (1977). *Scripts, plans, goals and understanding: An inquiry into human knowledge structures*. Hillsdale, NJ: Erlbaum Associates.

Schoeneman, T.J., & Rubanowitz, D.E. (1985). Attributions in the advice columns: Actors and observers, causes and reasons. *Personality and Social Psychology Bulletin*, *11*, 315–325.

Schouten, P.G.W., & Handelsman, M.M. (1987). Social basis of self-handicapping: The case of depression. *Personality and Social Psychology Bulletin*, *6*, 644–650.

Schulz, R., & Decker, S. (1985). Long-term adjustment to physical disability: The role of social support, perceived control, and self-blame. *Journal of Personality and Social Psychology*, *48*, 1162–1172.

Schunk, D.H. (1981). Modeling and attributional effects on children's achievement: A self-efficacy analysis. *Journal of Educational Psychology*, *73*, 93–105.

Schunk, D.H. (1982). Effects of effort attributional feedback in children's perceived self-efficacy and achievement. *Journal of Educational Psychology*, *74*, 548–556.

Schunk, D.H. (1983). Ability versus effort attributional feedback: Differential effects on self-efficacy and achievement. *Journal of Educational Psychology*, *75*, 848–852.

Schunk, D.H. (1984). Sequential attributional feedback and children's achievement behaviors. *Journal of Educational Psychology*, *76*, 1159–1169.

Schwartz, J.C., & Shaver, P. (1987). Emotions and emotion knowledge in interpersonal relations. In W. Jones & D. Perlman (Eds.), *Advances in personal relationships (Vol. 1)* (pp. 197–241). Greenwich, CT: JAI Press.

Scott, M.B., & Lyman, S. (1968). Accounts. *American Sociological Review, 33,* 46–62.

Seligman, M.E.P. (1973). Fall into helplessness. *Psychology Today,* pp. 43–48.

Seligman, M.E.P. (1975). *Helplessness: On depression, development, and death.* San Francisco: Freeman.

Seligman, M.E.P. (1980). A learned helplessness point of view. In L. Rehm (Ed.), *Behavior therapy for depression* (pp. 123–141). New York: Academic Press.

Seligman, M.E.P., Abramson, L.Y., Semmel, A., & Von Baeyer, C. (1979). Depressive attributional style. *Journal of Abnormal Psychology, 88,* 242–247.

Seligman, M.E.P., Castellon, C., Cacciola, J., Schulman, P., Luborsky, L., Ollove, M., & Downing, R. (1988). Explanatory style change during cognitive therapy for unipolar depression. *Journal of Abnormal Psychology, 97,* 13–18.

Seligman, M.E.P., & Maier, S.F. (1967). The alleviation of learned helplessness in the dog. *Journal of Experimental Psychology, 74,* 1–9.

Seligman, M.E.P., Maier, S.F., & Geer, J. (1968). The alleviation of learned helplessness in the dog. *Journal of Abnormal and Social Psychology, 73,* 256–262.

Seligman, M.E.P., Maier, S.F., & Solomon, R.L. (1971). Unpredictable and uncontrollable aversive events. In F.R. Brush (Ed.), *Aversive conditioning and learning* (pp. 347–400). New York: Academic Press.

Seligman, M.E.P., Peterson, C., Kaslow, N.J., Tanenbaum, R.L., Alloy, L.B., & Abramson, L.Y. (1984). Explanatory style and depressive symptoms among children. *Journal of Abnormal Psychology, 93,* 235–238.

Semin, G., & Manstead, A.S.R. (1983). *The accountability of conduct.* London: Academic Press.

Shapiro, D. (1965). *Neurotic styles.* New York: Basic Books.

Shaver, K.G. (1970). Defensive attribution: Effects of severity and relevance on the responsibility assigned for an accident. *Journal of Personality and Social Psychology, 14,* 101–113.

Shaver, K.G. (1975). *An introduction to attribution processes.* Cambridge: Winthrop.

Shaver, K.G. (1979). The land is fertile, but the farmers need a cooperative. *Contemporary Psychology, 24,* 680–682.

Shaver, K.G. (1985). *The attribution of blame: Causality, responsibility, and blameworthiness.* New York: Springer-Verlag.

Shaver, K.G., & Drown, D. (1986). On causality, responsibility, and self-blame: A theoretical note. *Journal of Personality and Social Psychology, 50,* 697–702.

Shaw, M.E., Bristoe, M.E., & Garcia-Esteve, J. (1968). A cross-cultural study of attribution of responsibility. *International Journal of Psychology, 3,* 51–60.

Shaw, M.E., & Iwawaki, S. (1972). Attribution of responsibility by Japanese and Americans as a function of age. *Journal of Cross-Cultural Psychology, 3,* 71–81.

Shaw, M.E., & Schneider, R.W. (1969). Intellectual competence as a variable in attribution of responsibility and assignment of sanctions. *Journal of Social Psychology, 78,* 31–39.

Shaw, M.E., & Sulzer, J.L. (1964). An empirical test of Heider's levels of attribution of responsibility. *Journal of Abnormal Social Psychology, 69,* 39–46.

Shields, N.M., & Hanneke, C.R. (1983). Attribution processes in violent relationships: Perceptions of violent husbands and their wives. *Journal of Applied Social Psychology, 13*, 515–527.

Shultz, T.R., & Butkowsky, I. (1977). Young children's use of the scheme for multiple sufficient causes in the attribution of real and hypothetical behavior. *Child Development, 48*, 464–469.

Shultz, T.R., Butkowsky, I., Pearce, J.W., & Shanfield, H. (1975). Development of schemes for the attribution of multiple psychological causes. *Developmental Psychology, 11*, 502–510.

Shultz, T.R., & Kestenbaum, N.R. (1985). Causal reasoning in children. *Annals of Child Development, 2*, 195–249.

Shultz, T.R., & Schleifer, M. (1983). Toward a refinement of attribution concepts. In J. Jaspers, F.D. Fincham, & M. Hewstone (Eds.), *Attribution theory and research: Conceptual, developmental, and social dimensions* (pp. 37–62). London: Academic Press.

Shultz, T.R., Schleifer, M., & Altman, I. (1981). Judgments of causation, responsibility, and punishment in cases of harm-doing. *Canadian Journal of Behavioral Science, 13*, 238–253.

Shultz, T.R., Wright, K., & Schleifer, M. (1986). Assignment of moral responsibility and punishment. *Child Development, 57*, 177–184.

Sigall, H., & Michela, J. (1976). I'll bet you say that to all the girls: Physical attractiveness and reactions to praise. *Journal of Personality, 44*, 611–626.

Sillars, A.L. (1981). Attributions and interpersonal conflict resolution. In J.H. Harvey, W.J. Ickes, R.F. Kidd (Eds.), *New directions in attribution research (Vol. 3)* (pp. 281–306). Hillsdale, NJ: Erlbaum Associates.

Silver, R.L., Boon, C., & Stones, M.H. (1983). Searching for meaning in misfortune: Making sense of incest. *Journal of Social Issues, 39*, 81–102.

Singerman, K.G., Borkovec, T.D., & Baron, R.S. (1976). Failure of a misattribution therapy manipulation with a clinically relevant target behavior. *Behavior Therapy, 7*, 306–313.

Skinner, B.F. (1957). *Verbal behavior.* New York: Appleton.

Smith, E.R. (1982). Beliefs, attributions, and evaluations: Nonhierarchical models of mediation in social cognition. *Journal of Personality and Social Psychology, 43*, 248–259.

Smith, E.R. (1984). Model of social inference processes. *Psychological Review, 91*, 392–413.

Smith, E.R., & Manard, B.B. (1980). Causal attributions and medical school admissions. *Personality and Soical Psychology Bulletin, 6*, 644–650.

Smith, E.R., & Miller, F.D. (1978). Limits on perception of cognitive processes: A reply to Nisbett and Wilson. *Psychological Review, 85*, 355–362.

Smith, E.R., & Miller, F.D. (1979). Salience and the cognitive mediation of attribution. *Journal of Personality and Social Psychology, 37*, 2240–2252.

Smith, M.C. (1975). Children's use of the multiple sufficient scheme in social perception. *Journal of Personality and Social Psychology, 32*, 737–747.

Smith, T.W., Snyder, C.R., & Handelsman, M.M. (1982). On the self-serving function of an academic wooden leg: Test anxiety as a self-handicapping strategy. *Journal of Personality and Social Psychology, 42*, 314–321.

Smith, T.W., Snyder, C.R., & Perkins, S.C. (1983). The self-serving function of hypochondriacal complaints: Physical symptoms as self-handicapping strategies. *Journal of Personality and Social Psychology*, *44*, 787–797.

Snyder, C.R., Smith, T.W., Augelli, R.W., & Ingram, R.E. (1985). On the self-serving function of social anxiety: Shyness as a self-handicapping strategy. *Journal of Personality and Social Psychology*, *48*, 970–980.

Snyder, M. (1976). Attribution and behavior: Social perception and social causation. In J.H. Harvey, W.J. Ickes, & R.F. Kidd (Eds.), *New directions in attribution research (Vol. 1)* (pp. 53–72). Hillsdale, NJ: Erlbaum Associates.

Snyder, M.L., Stephan, W.G., & Rosenfield, D. (1978). Attributional egotism. In J.H. Harvey, W.J. Ickes, & R.F. Kidd (Eds.), *New directions in attribution research (Vol. 2)* (pp. 91–117). Hillsdale, NJ: Erlbaum Associates.

Snyder, M.L., & Wicklund, R.A. (1981). Attribute ambiguity. In J.H. Harvey, W.J. Ickes, & R.F. Kidd (Eds.), *New directions in attribution research (Vol. 3)* (pp. 199–224). Hillsdale, NJ: Erlbaum Associates.

Sohn, D. (1977). Affect-generating powers of effort and ability self attributions of academic success and failure. *Journal of Educational Psychology*, *69*, 500–505.

Solomon, S. (1978). Measuring dispositional and situational attributions. *Personality and Social Psychology Bulletin*, *4*, 589–593.

Sonne, J.L., & Janoff, D. (1979). The effect of treatment of attributions on the maintenance of weight reduction: A replication and extension. *Cognitive Theory and Research*, *3*, 389–397.

Spring, B., Chiodo, J., & Bowen, D.J. (1987). The social–clinical–psychobiology interface: Implications for health psychology. *Journal of Social and Clinical Psychology*, *5*, 1–7.

Srull, T.K. (1981). Person memory: Some tests of associatve storage and retrieval models. *Journal of Experimental Social Psychology*, *7*, 440–462.

Stephan, W.G., & Gollwitzer, P.M. (1981). Affect as a mediator of attributional egotism. *Journal of Experimental Social Psychology*, *17*, 442–458.

Stern, R.M., Botto, R.W., & Herrick, C.D. (1972). Behavioral and physiological effects of false heart rate feedback: A replication and extension. *Psychophysiology*, *9*, 21–29.

Storms, M.D. (1973). Videotape and the attribution process: Reversing actors' and observers' points of view. *Journal of Personality and Social Psychology*, *27*, 165–175.

Storms, M.D., Denney, D.R., McCaul, K.D., & Lowery, C.R. (1979). Treating insomnia. In J.H. Frieze, D. Bar-Tal, & J.S. Carroll (Eds.), *New approaches to social problems* (pp. 151–167). San Francisco: Jossey Bass.

Storms, M.D., & McCaul, K.D. (1975). *Stuttering, attribution, and exacerbation.* Unpublished manuscript, University of Kansas, Lawrence.

Storms, M.D., & McCaul, K.D. (1976). Attribution processes and emotional exacerbation of dysfunctional behavior. In J.H. Harvey, W.J. Ickes, & R.F. Kidd (Eds.), *New directions in attribution research (Vol. 1)* (pp. 143–164). Hillsdale, NJ: Erlbaum Associates.

Storms, M.D., & Nisbett, R.E. (1970). Insomnia and the attribution process. *Journal of Personality and Social Psychology*, *16*, 319–328.

Strube, M. (1985). Attributional style and the Type A coronary-prone behavior pattern. *Journal of Personality and Social Psychology*, *49*, 500–509.

Strube, M.J. (1987). A self-appraisal model of the Type A behavior pattern. In

R. Hogen & W. Jones (Eds.), *Perspectives in personality: Theory, measurement, and interpersonal dynamics* (Vol. 2) (pp. 201–250). Greenwich, CT: JAI Press.

Strube, M.J. (1988). Performance attributions and the Type A behavior pattern: Causal sources versus causal dimensions. *Personality and Social Psychology Bulletin, 14*, 709–721.

Strube, M.J., & Boland, S.M. (1986). Post-performance attributions and task persistence among Type A and B individuals: A clarification. *Journal of Personality and Social Psychology, 50*, 413–420.

Stryker, S., & Gottlieb, A. (1981). Attribution theory and symbolic interactionism: A comparison. In J.H. Harvey, W.J. Ickes, & R.F. Kidd (Eds.), *New directions in attribution research (Vol. 3)* (pp. 425–458). Hillsdale, NJ: Erlbaum Associates.

Surra, C.A. (1985). Courtship types: Variations in interdependence between partners and social networks. *Journal of Personality and Social Psychology, 49*, 357–375.

Surra, C.A. (1988). *Turning point coding manual III.* Unpublished manuscript, Division of Family Studies, University of Arizona, Tucson.

Surra, C.A., Arizzi, P., & Asmussen, L.A. (1988). The association between reasons for commitment and the development and outcome of marital relationships. *Journal of Social and Personal Relationships, 5*, 47–63.

Sushinsky, L.S., & Bootzin, R.R. (1970). Cognitive desensitization as a model of systematic desensitization. *Behavior Research and Therapy, 8*, 29–33.

Sweeney, P.D., Anderson, K., & Bailey, S. (1986). Attributional style in depression: A meta-analytic review. *Journal of Personality and Soical Psychology, 50*, 974–991.

Tait, R., & Silver, R.C. (in press). Coming to terms with major negative life events. In J.S. Uleman & J.A. Bargh (Eds.), *Unintended thought: The limits of awareness, intention, and control.* New York: Guilford Press.

Taylor, S.E. (1981). The interface of cognitive and social psychology. In J.H. Harvey (Ed.), *Cognition, social behavior, and the environment* (pp. 189–212). Hillsdale, NJ: Erlbaum Associates.

Taylor, S.E., & Fiske, S.T. (1978). Salience, attention, and attribution: Top of the head phenomena. In L. Berkowitz (Ed.), *Advances in experimental social psychology (Vol. 11)* (pp. 249–288). New York: Academic Press.

Taylor, S.E., Lichtman, R.R., & Wood, J.V. (1984). Attributions, beliefs about control, and adjustment to breast cancer. *Journal of Personality and Social Psychology, 46*, 489–502.

Taylor, S.E., Wood, J.V., & Lichtman, R.R. (1983). It could be worse: Selective evaluation as a response to victimization. *Journal of Social Issues, 39*, 19–40.

Tennen, H., Affleck, G., & Gershman, K. (1986). Self-blame among parents of infants with perinatal complications: The role of self-protective motives. *Journal of Personality and Soical Psychology, 50*, 690–696.

Tennen, H., & Herzberger, S. (1987). Depression, self-esteem, and the absence of self-protective attributional biases. *Journal of Personality and Social Psychology, 52*, 72–80.

Tepper, M.E., & Powers, S. (1984). Prediction of high school algebra achievement with attributional, motivational, and achievement measures. *Perceptual and Motor Skills, 59*, 120–122.

Tetlock, P.E. (1980). Explaining teacher explanations of pupil performance: A self-presentation interpretation. *Social Psychology Quarterly, 43*, 283–290.

Tetlock, P.E. (1985). Accountability: A social check on the fundamental attribution error. *Social Psychology Quarterly*, *48*, 227–236.

Tetlock, P.E., & Levi, A. (1982). Attribution bias: On the inconclusiveness of the cognition–motivation debate. *Journal of Experimental Social Psychology*, *18*, 68–88.

Tharp, R.G. (1963). Psychological patterning in marriage. *Psychological Bulletin*, *60*, 97–117.

Thibaut, J.W., & Riecken, H.W. (1955). Some determinants and consequences of the perception of social causality. *Journal of Personality*, *24*, 113–133.

Thompson, S.C., & Kelley, H.H. (1981). Judgments of responsibility for activities in close relationships. *Journal of Personality and Social Psychology*, *41*, 469–477.

Timko, C., & Janoff-Bulman, R. (1985). Attributions, invulnerability, and psychological adjustment: The case of breast cancer. *Health Psychology*, *4*, 521–544.

Trope, Y. (1986). Identification and inferential processes in dispositional attribution. *Psychological Review*, *93*, 239–257.

Tucker, J.A., Vuchinich, R.E., & Sobell, M.B. (1981). Alcohol consumption as a self-handicapping strategy. *Journal of Abnormal Psychology*, *90*, 220–230.

Turnquist, D.C., Harvey, J.H., & Andersen, B.L. (1988). Attributions and adjustment to life-threatening illness. *British Journal of Clinical psychology*, *27*, 55–65.

Valins, S. (1966). Cognitive effects of false heart-rate feedback. *Journal of Personality and Social Psychology*, *4*, 400–408.

Valins, S., & Nisbett, R.E. (1972). Attribution processes in the development and treatment of emotional disorders. In E.E. Jones, D.E. Kanouse, H.H. Kelley, R.E. Nisbett, S. Valins, & B. Weiner (Eds.), *Attribution: Perceiving the causes of behavior* (pp. 137–150). Morristown NJ: General Learning Press.

Valins, S., & Ray, A. (1967). Effects of cognitive desensitization on avoidance behavior. *Journal of Personality and Social Psychology*, *20*, 239–250.

Vinokur, A., & Ajzen, I. (1982). Relative importance of prior and immediate events: A causal primacy effect. *Journal of Personality and Soical Psychology*, *42*, 820–829.

Wachtler, J., & Counselman, E. (1981). When increasing liking for a communicator decreases opinion change: An attribution analysis of attractiveness. *Journal of Experimental Social Psychology*, *17*, 386–395.

Walster, E. (1966). Assignment of responsibility for an accident. *Journal of Personality and Social Psychology*, *3*, 73–79.

Watson, D. (1982). The actor and the observer: How are their perceptions of causality divergent? *Psychological Bulletin*, *92*, 682–700.

Watzlawick, P., Beavin, J., & Jackson, D. (1967). *Pragmatics of human communication: A study of interactional patterns, pathologies, and paradoxes.* New York: W.W. Norton.

Weary, G. (1979). Self-serving attributional biases: Perceptual or response distortions? *Journal of Personality and Social Psychology*, *37*, 1418–1420.

Weary, G. (1980). Affect and egotism as mediators of bias in causal attributions. *Journal of Personality and Social Psychology*, *38*, 348–357.

Weary, G., & Arkin, R.M. (1981). Attributional self-presentation. In J.H. Harvey, W.J. Ickes, & R.F. Kidd (Eds.), *New directions in attribution research (Vol. 3)* (pp. 225–247). Hillsdale, NJ: Erlbaum Associates.

Weary, G., Harvey, J.H., Schweiger, P., Olson, C.T., Perloff, R., Pritchard, S.

(1982). Self-presentation and the moderation of self-serving attributional biases. *Social Cognition, 1*, 140–159.

Weary, G., & Mirels, H.L. (Eds.). (1982). *Integration of clinical and social psychology*. New York: Oxford University Press.

Weary Bradley, G. (1978). Self-serving biases in the attribution process: A reexamination of the fact or fiction question. *Journal of Personality and Social Psychology, 36*, 56–71.

Weber, A.L., Harvey, J.H., & Stanley, M.A. (1978). The nature and motivations of accounts for failed relationships. In R. Burnett, P. McGhee, & D.C. Clarke (Eds.), *Accounting for relationships* (pp. 114–133). London: Methuen.

Weiner, B. (Ed.). (1974). *Achievement motivation and attribution theory*. Morristown, NJ: General Learning Press.

Weiner, B. (1977). Attribution and affect: Comments on Sohn's critique. *Journal of Educational Psychology, 69*, 506–511.

Weiner, B. (1979). A theory of motivation for some classroom experiences. *Journal of Educational Psychology, 71*, 3–25.

Weiner, B. (1980). The role of affect in rational attributional approaches to human motivation and emotion. *Educational Researcher, 9*, 4–11.

Weiner, B. (1985). An attributional theory of achievement motivation and emotion. *Psychological Review, 92*, 548–573.

Weiner, B. (1986). *An attributional theory of motivation and emotion*. New York: Springer-Verlag.

Weiner, B., & Brown, J. (1984). All's well that ends. *Journal of Educational Psychology, 76*, 169–171.

Weiner, B., Frieze, I.H., Kukla, A., Reed, L., Rest, S., & Rosenbaum, R.M. (1971). *Perceiving the causes of success and failure*. Morristown, NJ: General Learning Press.

Weiner, B., Frieze, I., Kukla, A., Reed, L., Rest, S., & Rosenbaum, R.M. (1972). Perceiving the causes of success and failure. In E.E. Jones, D.E. Kanouse H.H. Kelley, R.E. Nisbett, S. Valins, & B. Weiner (Eds.), *Attribution: Perceiving the causes of behavior* (pp. 95–120). Morristown, NJ: General Learning Press.

Weiner, B., Graham, S., & Chandler, C. (1982). Causal antecedents of pity, anger, and guilt. *Personality and Social Psychology Bulletin, 8*, 226–232.

Weiner, B., Heckhausen, H., Meyer, W.U., & Cook, R.E. (1972). Causal ascriptions and achievement behavior: A conceptual analysis of effort and reanalysis of locus of control. *Journal of Personality and Social Psychology, 21*, 239–248.

Weiner, B., & Kukla, A. (1970). An attributional analysis of achievement motivation. *Journal of Personality and Social Psychology, 15*, 1–20.

Weiner, B., Nierenberg, R., & Goldstein, M. (1976). Social learning (LOC) versus attributional (causal stability) interpretations of expectancy of success. *Journal of Personality, 44*, 52–68.

Weiner, B., Russell, D., & Lerman, D. (1978). Affective consequences of caual ascriptions. In J.H. Harvey, W.J. Ickes, & R.F. Kidd (Eds.), *New directions in attribution research (Vol. 2)* (pp. 59–90). Hillsdale, NJ: Erlbaum Associates.

Weiner, B., Russell, D., & Lerman, D. (1979). The cognition–emotion process in achievement-related contexts. *Journal of Personality and Social Psychology, 37*, 1211–1220.

Weiss, R.S. (1975). *Marital separation*. New York: Basic Books.

Wells, D., & Shultz, T.R. (1980). Developmental distinctions between behavior and judgment in the operation of the discounting principle. *Child Development, 51*, 1307–1310.

Wells, G.L., & Harvey, J.H. (1977). Do people use consensus information in making causal attributions? *Journal of Personality and Social Psychology, 35*, 279–293.

Wells, G.L., Petty, R.E., Harkins, S.G., Kagehiro, D., & Harvey J.H. (1977). Anticipated discussion of interpretation eliminates actor–observer differences in the attribution of causality. *Sociometry, 46*, 247–253.

Wells, G.L., & Ronis, D.L. (1982). Discounting and augmentation: Is there something special about the number of causes? *Personality and Social Psychology Bulletin, 8*, 566–572.

Whalen, C.K., & Henker, B. (1976). Psychostimulants and children: A review and analysis. *Psychological Bulletin, 83*, 1113–1130.

White, G.L., & Kight, T.D. (1984). Misattribution of arousal and attraction: Effects of salience of explanations for arousal. *Journal of Experimental Social Psychology, 20*, 55–64.

White, P. (1980). Limitations on verbal reports of internal states: A refutation of Nisbett and Wilson and of Bem. *Psychological Review, 87*, 105–112.

Wilder, D. (1978a). Effects of predictability on units of perception and attraction. *Personality and Social Psychology Bulletin, 4*, 281–284.

Wilder, D. (1978b). Predictability of behaviors, goals, and unit of perception. *Personality and Social Psychology Bulletin, 4*, 604–607.

Wilson, T.D. (1985). Strangers to ourselves: The origins and accuracy of beliefs about one's own mental states. In J.H. Harvey & G. Weary (Eds.), *Attribution: Basic issues and applications* (pp. 9–36). Orlando, FL: Academic Press.

Wilson, T.D., Hull, J.G., & Johnson, J. (1981). Awareness and self-perception: Verbal reports on internal states. *Journal of Personality and Social Psychology, 40*, 53–71.

Wilson, T.D., & Linville, P.W. (1982). Improving the academic performance of college freshmen: Attribution therapy revisited. *Journal of Personality and Social Psychology, 42*, 367–376.

Wilson, T.D., & Linville, P.W. (1985). Improving the performance of college freshmen with attributional techniques. *Journal of Personality and Social Psychology, 49*, 287–293.

Wimer, S., & Kelley, H.H. (1982). An investigation of the dimensions of causal attribution. *Journal of Personality and Social Psychology, 43*, 1142–1162.

Wong, P.T.P., & Weiner, B. (1981). When people ask "why" questions, and the heuristics of attributional search. *Journal of Personality and Social Psychology, 40*, 650–663.

Wood, W., & Eagly, A.H. (1981). Stages in the analysis of persuasive messages: The role of causal attributions and message comprehension. *Journal of Personality and Social Psychology, 40*, 246–259.

Wortman, C.B. (1983). Coping with victimization: Conclusions and implications for future research. *Journal of Social Issues, 35*, 120–155.

Wortman, C.B., & Brehm, J.W. (1975). Responses to uncontrollable outcomes: An integration of reactance theory and the learned helplessness model. In L. Berkowitz (Ed.), *Advances in experimental social psychology (Vol. 8)* (pp. 277–336). New York: Academic Press.

Wortman, C.B., & Dunkel-Schetter, C. (1979). Interpersonal relationships and cancer: A theoretical analysis. *Journal of Social Issues*, *35*, 120–155.

Wyer, R.S., & Carlston, D.E. (1979). *Social cognition, inference and attribution*. Hillsdale, NJ: Erlbaum Associates.

Yarkin, K.L., Harvey, J.H., & Bloxom, B.M. (1981). Cognitive sets, attribution, and social interaction. *Journal of Personality and Social Psychology*, *41*, 243–252.

Zillmann, D. (1978). Attribution and misattribution of excitatory reactions. In J.H. Harvey, W.J. Ickes, R.F. Kidd (Eds.), *New direction in attribution research (Vol. 2)* (pp. 335–370). Hillsdale, NJ: Erlbaum Associates.

Zillmann, D. (1983). Transfer of excitation in emotional behavior. In J.T. Cacioppo & R.E. Petty (Eds.), *Social psychophysiology* (pp. 88–112). New York: Guilford.

Zillmann, D., & Cantor, J.R. (1976). Effect of timing of information about mitigating circumstances on emotional responses to provocation and retaliatory behavior. *Journal of Experimental Social Psychology*, *12*, 38–55.

Zuckerman, M. (1978). Use of consensus information in prediction of behavior. *Journal of Experimental Social Psychology*, *14*, 163–171.

Zuckerman, M. (1979). Attribution of success and failure revisited, or: The motivational bias is alive and well in attribution theory. *Journal of Personality*, *47*, 245–287.

Zuckerman, M., Eghrari, H., & Lambrecht, M.R. (1986). Attributions as inferences and explanations: Conjunction effects. *Journal of Personality and Social Psychology*, *51*, 1144–1153.

Zuckerman, M., & Evans, S. (1984). Schematic approach to the attributional processing of actions and occurrences. *Journal of Personality and Social Psychology*, *47*, 469–478.

Zuckerman, M., & Feldman, L.S. (1984). Actions and occurrences in attribution theory. *Journal of Personality and Social Psychology*, *46*, 541–550.

Author Index

Subject Index